by James Mil

Instant Pot
Gluten Free
40 Cookbook
Healthy, Easy, Delicious & Nutritious Gluten-Free Recipes

Editor: Jeff Miller
Design: Steven Gunzler
Proofreader: Helen Stephanie
Production manager: Irene Shuman

Text Copyright © James Miller

Legal & Disclaimer

Contents

Introduction

Nowadays, we never have enough time for anything. We are always in a hurry to leave our office or finish every day work at home. Being at home or office, the time is always an asset in this modern lifestyle. Also we cannot neglect the need of consuming wholesome foods as a well-balanced nutrition is very important to stay healthy.

Instant Pot takes care of both your everyday nutritional needs and time crunch by making food in minutes. You can imagine Instant Pot as a cooking robot, which makes delicious meals for you in minutes. Instant pot frees a lot of your time by doing almost all cooking work so that you can spend more time with your family.

What Exactly Is Instant Pot?

Instant Pot is your multi-purpose kitchen partner that makes a cooking process fun and effortless for you. It is a modern revolutionary invention and a good investment, if you buy it, it will take care of your all modern cooking needs. You can also cook food in batches, freeze them, and simply heat up later. Different Instant Pot models come in different sizes and with many programmable features. All models come with basic cooking features and basic settings.

This revolutionary technology helps in sealing most of the nutrients in the food. Instant pot is a multi-functional kitchen invention that performs all the functions that you can perform using an electric pressure cooker, slow cooker, steamer or warming pot. In short, it is one-in-all cooking appliance.

How Instant Pot Works?

With Instant Pot, you simply need to place all the ingredients into the pot and it is done. This modern appliance uses pressured steam to help you cook delicious meals. It cooks added ingredients, be it vegetables, grains, rice, spices, liquid or anything else, Instant pot cooks added ingredients with extremely high-pressure steam and that is the reason for its real quick cooking cycle. It cooks most of your favorite cuisines in a matter of minutes without the need of your constant attention.

1. You need to first plug your instant pot in a power socket and then open its top lid.
2. Now you just have to add recipe ingredients in the pot and then close the lid.
3. Now you have to set cooking time as instructed in recipe and then it's done.
4. Instant Pot slowly builds pressure and cooks the food for you.
5. After the cooking time is over, you have to release inside pressure, open the lid and enjoy your hot meal.

NPR (Natural Pressure Release)
This setting means that you let Instant Pot naturally release pressure. Leave the vent valve alone until it releases all inside pressure by its own.
QPR (Quick Pressure Release)
This means that you manually release the pressure quickly by twisting the vent valve. It releases pressure in quick time. Open the valve slowly for a while until the force reduces.

Instant Pot: Modern & Smart Cooking Settings

Instant pot provides you with the most modern cooking functions and can cook anything for you with many pre-set cooking modules. Following are common settings for a convenient cooking experience.

Keep Warm/Cancel

With this function you can cancel any program that has been previously; it puts the cooker in standby and keeps it warm for some time.

In a manual way

With this setting, you can manually set your own pressure and cook time.

Rice

With this function, your Instant pot works as a rice cooker. With this setting, you can easily prepare various rice-based meals and other cuisines. The default option for this setting is automatic and cooks rice at low pressure. You can use "Adjust" setting to set your choice of time.

Slow Cook

With this function your Instant pot works as a rice cooker, which can cook to up to 40 hours, but the default setting is for 4 hours.

Poultry

With this setting you can easily prepare meals with poultry and the default is set at high pressure for 15 minutes.

Bean/Chili

With this setting you can easily prepare chili or beans. The default is high pressure for 30 minutes.

Multigrain

With this setting you can easily prepare a mixture of grains such as brown rice, beans, wild rice etc. The default option for this setting is 40 minutes of high pressure.

Cake & Egg

This setting is to cook a variety of cake and egg based recipes.

Porridge

With this setting you can easily prepare oatmeal or porridge of various grains. This default option makes high pressure for 20 minutes.

Meat/Stew

With this setting you can easily prepare meats or stew and the default is set at high pressure for 35 minutes.

Soup

With this setting you can easily prepare a variety of broths and soups. The default is set for 30 minutes of high pressure.

Yogurt

The default of this setting is 8 hours of cooking time to make various types of yogurts. You can use "Adjust" to increase or decrease time.

Sauté

This setting is for sautéing ingredient with the lid open; this function is for browning, sautéing or simmering of added ingredients usually oil, onions, garlic, etc.

Steam

You can use this function for steaming seafood, veggies or reheating foods. The default is 10 minutes of high-pressure cooking.

Benefits of Cooking with Instant Pot

There are many reasons why Instant Pot is being called modern kitchen revolution. It makes your life easy and provides you with a healthy food every day to improve your lifestyle.

Saves Time & Energy

Instant pot takes a few minutes to cook food as compared to other cooking methods. It works particularly well with dried ingredients including legumes, beans, pulses and grains. With Instant Pot, you can skip pre-soaking them for 2 to 12 hours prior to cooking time as you can directly add them in the pot and it will cook them for you without the need for soaking.

All you need to do is to add the recommended amount of liquids and other ingredients. At high pressure, you can cook legumes, beans, pulses and grains in less than 30 minutes.

Maintains Nutritional Values

Unlike many other cooking methods, which require you to fully immerse the vegetables and other ingredients under the water in order to cook them, instant pot needs just enough water to cook your vegetables, meats, grains and much more. It maintains high pressure steam levels and preserves nutritional values. This technique prevents essential vitamins, minerals, proteins and anti-oxidants from being washed away.

Cooking Convenience

Instant Pot comes with 12-key functions which include poultry, rice, bean/chili, meat/ stew, soup, multi-grain, steam, porridges, and other control keys. Each cooking setting has certain pre-set specifications for pressure and time. Either you can cook at pre-set time and pressure, or you can easily adjust time as per your convenience.

Removes Harmful Bacteria & Fungus

The water level is heated in Instant Pot at a very high temperature where a lot of diseases causing by micro-organisms are killed off. It kills harmful bacteria and fungus from grains and vegetables to serve you with healthy meals every time.

Instant Pot & Gluten-Free Cooking

If you are having gluten intolerance due to your body's inability to process gluten containing ingredients then that does not mean that you can't replace your favorite foods. There are delicious and nutritious replacements available for most of the gluten-containing ingredients. Sever gluten sensitivity can also lead to celiac disease. Pasta, bread, noodles, crackers, etc. are commonly used ingredients with gluten and must be avoided for people with gluten sensitivity.

Healthy Gluten Free Swaps

Ingredient	Healthy Gluten-Free Swap
All-purpose flour	Gluten-free flour
Flour tortilla	Corn tortilla
Crackers	Gluten-free crackers
Bread crumbs	Gluten-free oats or almond meal breadcrumbs
Rice	Cauliflower rice
Lasagna	Zucchini lasagna
Hamburger buns	Portobello zucchini buns
Pasta	Zucchini pasta
Hash browns	Spaghetti squash

Instant pot is designed to prepare wholesome gluten-free recipes at home and enjoy their wholesomeness every day. Instant pot lets you allow cooking gluten-free cuisines in real quick time along with preserving their rich nutritional content. When it comes to Instant Pot cooking, your options are not limited when you are following a gluten-free diet regimen. Every day, new and healthy recipes are being invented for Instant Pot to celebrate 100% gluten-free diet.

This book provides you with 40 nutritious gluten-free recipes to prepare in your Instant Pot so you can enjoy tasty breakfast, lunch, dinner and dessert recipes with your whole family. This book covers popular gluten-free ingredients to get the best flavors of your meal time. These gluten free ingredients are healthy swaps for commonly used ingredients containing gluten. A versatile collection of 40 recipes has everything to offer to enjoy your favorite cuisines.

Let's start preparing wholesome meals with Instant Pot in real quick time and make it a memorable cooking experience.

Chapter 1:
Wholesome Breakfast Recipes

Wholesome Cherry Rice Breakfast

Prep Time: 8-10 min. | Serves: 2-3

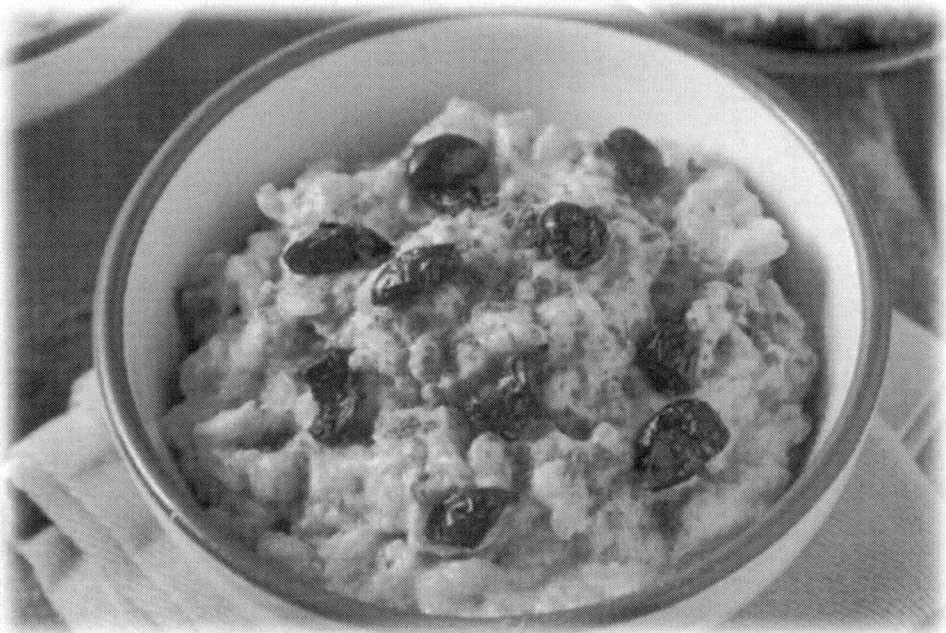

Directions:

- Switch on your instant pot. Make sure that your kitchen platform is clean and dry.
- Select "Saute" setting from various available options.
- Open the pot and add some butter and rice; heat for 4-5 minutes, stirring.
- Add sugar, apples, and spices, and stir again.
- Add milk and apple juice; stir and mix.
- Make sure to lock the lid properly after closing the pot. Also ensure to seal the valve.
- Select "Manual" setting from various available options. Adjust cooking time to 6 minutes.
- Allow the mixture to cook under pressure until the timer reads zero.
- Turn off and press "Cancel" setting.
- Open the pot and transfer the mixture to a serving bowl.
- Add dried cherries, stir and serve hot!

Ingredients:

1 ½ cups of Arborio rice, gluten free
3 cups of milk
2 tbs. of butter
1 cup of apple juice
1 ½ tsp. of cinnamon
½ cup of dried cherries
2 apples, cored, chopped
1/3 cup of brown sugar
¼ tsp. of salt

Nutritional Value (Per Serving):

Calories – 430 | Fat – 10g | Carbohydrate – 38g | Fiber – 3g | Protein – 7g

Creamy Sausage Frittata

Prep Time: 30-40 min. | Serves: 3-4

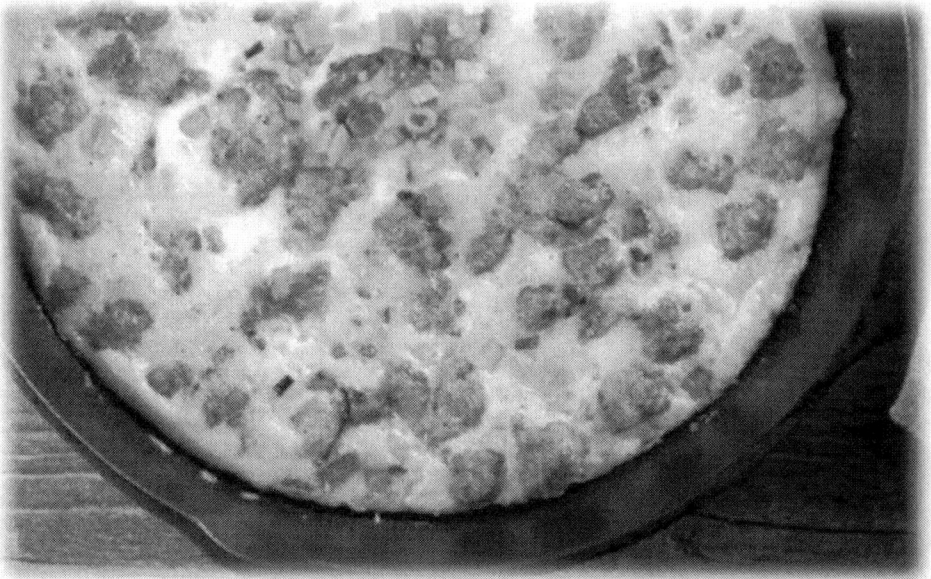

Directions:

- Switch on your instant pot. Make sure that your kitchen platform is clean and dry.
- Pour some water in the pot. Arrange a trivet inside.
- Lightly grease a 6-inch baking dish with butter.
- In a bowl of medium size, thoroughly mix eggs and sour cream. Add sausage, cheese, scallions, pepper and salt; mix well.
- Pour the mixture into a buttered pan.
- Cover the pan with foil and place on the trivet.
- Make sure to lock the lid properly after closing the pot. Also ensure to seal the valve.
- Select "Manual" setting from various available options. Adjust cooking time to 15-17 minutes.
- Allow the mixture to cook under pressure until the timer reads zero.
- Turn off and press "Cancel" setting.
- Open the pot and serve hot!

Ingredients:

2 tbs. of sour cream
½ cup of cooked sausage, crumbled
¼ cup of cheddar cheese, grated
1 ½ cups of water
1 tbs. of butter
4 eggs, beaten
2 scallions, chopped
Pepper and salt to taste

Nutritional Value (Per Serving):

Calories – 281 | Fat – 12g | Carbohydrate – 4g | Fiber – 0g | Protein – 16g

Pancetta Egg Morning

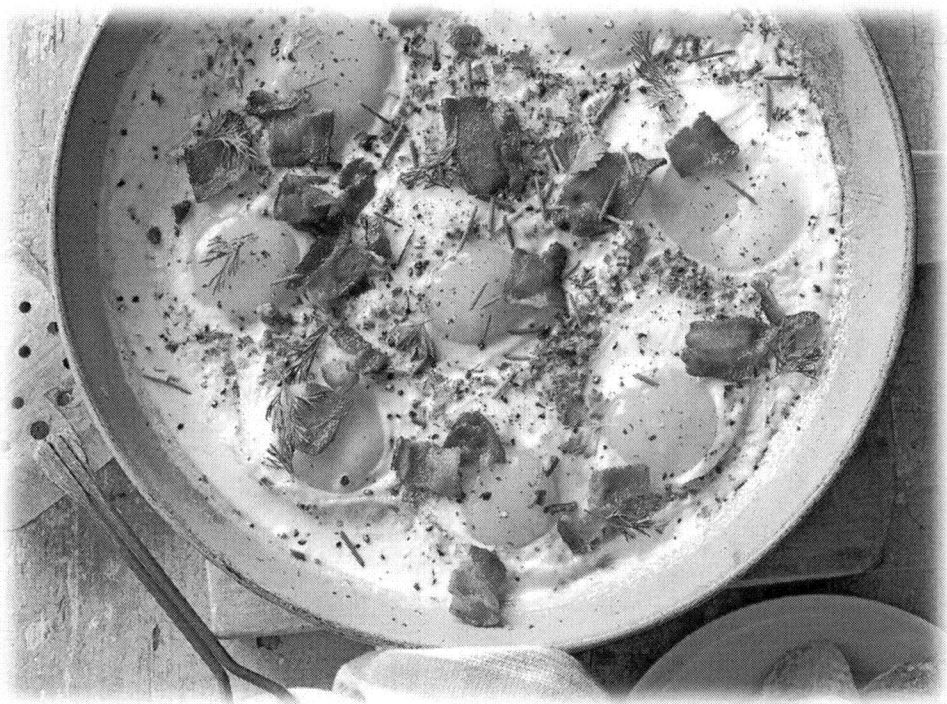

Directions:

- Preheat an oven to 450 F. Line a baking sheet with a parchment paper.
- In a bowl of medium size, thoroughly mix the egg whites, pancetta, onions, and cheese. Stir well.
- Switch on your instant pot. Make sure that your kitchen platform is clean and dry.
- Select "Saute" setting from various available options.
- Open the pot and add the egg mixture; heat for 1 minutes to cook well.
- Add cooked mixture into the parchment paper.
- Bake for 3-4 minutes. Remove from the oven and add the egg yolks.
- Bake for another 3 minutes and serve hot!

Ingredients:

2 tbs. of green onions, chopped
2 eggs, large
2 pancetta pieces, browned and crumbled
½ cup of Mexican cheese, shredded

Nutritional Value (Per Serving):

Calories – 273 | Fat – 21g | Carbohydrate – 2g | Fiber – 0g | Protein – 18g

Classic Milk Oats

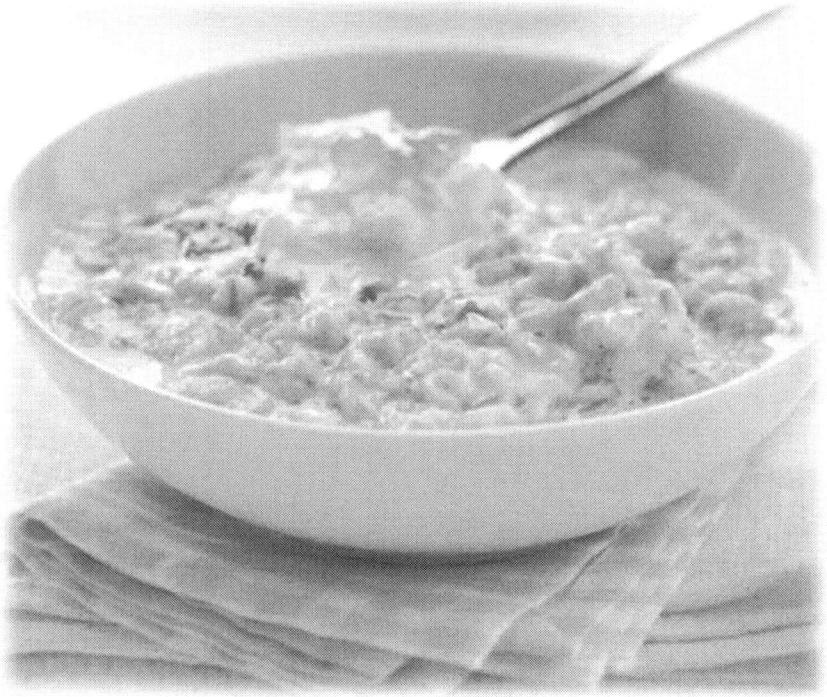

Directions:

- Switch on your instant pot. Make sure that your kitchen platform is clean and dry.
- Open the lid and gradually add all the above mentioned ingredients in the pot.
- Make sure to lock the lid properly after closing the pot. Also ensure to seal the valve.
- Select "Manual" setting from various available options. Adjust cooking time to 10 minutes.
- Allow the mixture to cook under pressure until the timer reads zero.
- Turn off and press "Cancel" setting.
- Let inside pressure to release naturally; it will take 8-10 minutes for pressure release.
- Open the pot and transfer the mixture to a serving bowl.
- Pour milk over the top, stir well; serve with your favorite dried fruit and nuts.

Ingredients:

½ cup of steel-cut oats, gluten free
2 cups of water
A pinch of salt
1 tbs. of oil
Milk as needed
2 tbs. of dried fruit and nuts

Nutritional Value (Per Serving):

Calories – 182 | Fat – 8g | Carbohydrate – 24.5g | Fiber – 3g | Protein – 4g

Bacon Cheesy Muffins

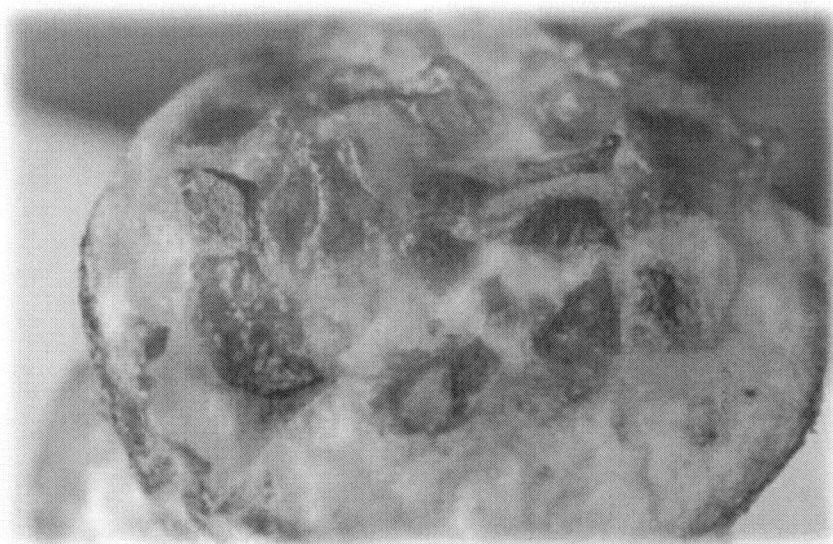

Directions:

- Switch on your instant pot. Make sure that your kitchen platform is clean and dry.
- Pour some water in the pot. Arrange a trivet inside.
- In a bowl of medium size, thoroughly mix eggs and pepper seasoning.
- Take an onion, cheese, and bacon; divide it between four silicone muffin tins.
- Divide the egg mixture between the tins.
- Add the muffins over the trivet.
- Make sure to lock the lid properly after closing the pot. Also ensure to seal the valve.
- Select "Manual" setting from various available options. Adjust cooking time to 8 minutes.
- Allow the mixture to cook under pressure until the timer reads zero.
- Turn off and press "Cancel" setting.
- Open the pot.
- Serve with green onion and tomato on top.

Ingredients:

1 green onion, chopped
4 tbs. of cheddar, shredded
4 eggs
4 slices of cooked bacon, crumbled
¼ tsp. of lemon pepper seasoning
1 ½ cups of water
Cherry tomatoes, make quarters

Nutritional Value (Per Serving):

Calories – 112 | Fat – 8g | Carbohydrate – 2.5g | Fiber – 0g | Protein – 8g

Jalapeno Egg Hash

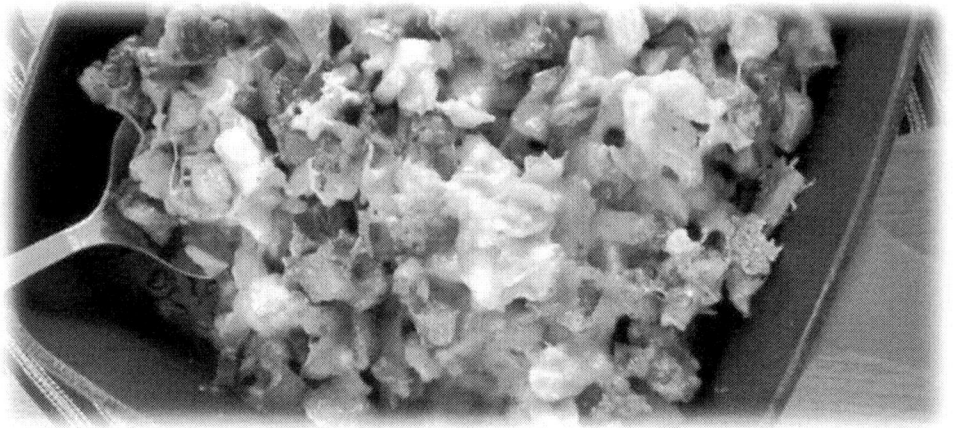

Directions:

- Switch on your instant pot. Make sure that your kitchen platform is clean and dry.
- Pour some water in the pot. Arrange a trivet inside.
- Add the potatoes to a bowl and place the bowl over the trivet.
- Make sure to lock the lid properly after closing the pot. Also ensure to seal the valve.
- Select "Manual" setting from various available options. Adjust cooking time to 2 minutes.
- Allow the mixture to cook under pressure until the timer reads zero.
- Turn off and press "Cancel" setting.
- Open the pot and drain water; set the cooked potatoes aside.
- Select "Saute" setting from various available options.
- Add butter and onions; heat for 2 minutes to cook well and soften.
- Add cilantro, pepper, taco seasoning, and the potatoes; combine well.
- Make a well in the center of the mixture, and break eggs over.
- Make sure to lock the lid properly after closing the pot. Also ensure to seal the valve.
- Select "Manual" setting from various available options. Adjust cooking time to 1 minute.
- Sprinkle some more cilantro on top. Serve hot!

Ingredients:

2 eggs
1 tbs. of cilantro, chopped
1 cup of potatoes, peeled, cubed
1 tsp. of taco seasoning
½ cup of diced onion
2 tbs. of butter
1 tbs. of bacon, cooked and chopped
1 jalapeno pepper, sliced
1 cup of water

Nutritional Value (Per Serving):
Calories – 394 | Fat – 19g | Carbohydrate – 42g | Fiber – 5g | Protein – 12g

Potato Onion Frittata

Prep Time: 35-40 min. | Serves: 3-4

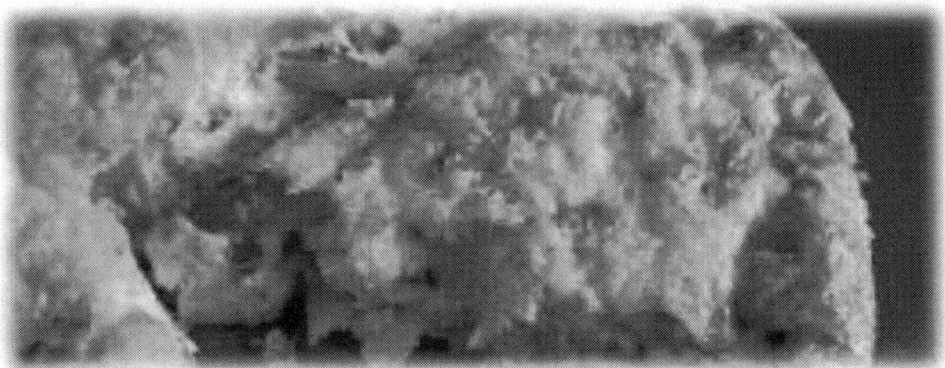

Directions:

- Switch on your instant pot. Make sure that your kitchen platform is clean and dry.
- Select "Saute" setting from various available options.
- Open the pot and add some oil and potato slices; heat for 3-4 minutes to cook well and soften.
- Flip and cook other side for 2 minutes; set aside.
- Add onion and cook for 2 minutes; now add bell pepper and cook for 2 minutes; remove from pot. Select Cancel.
- Pour some water in the pot. Arrange a trivet inside and add the mixture over the trivet.
- Butter a 6-inch baking dish. Beat eggs in a medium size bowl and add cream, pepper and salt to taste; combine well.
- Arrange half of potatoes, bell pepper, and onion in the baking dish.
- Pour half egg mixture on top and sprinkle with cheese. Repeat again.
- Cover with a foil, add the dish on a steam rack.
- Make sure to lock the lid properly after closing the pot. Also ensure to seal the valve.
- Select "Manual" setting from various available options. Adjust cooking time to 16 minutes.
- Allow the mixture to cook under pressure until the timer reads zero.
- Turn off and press "Cancel" setting.
- Serve hot!

Ingredients:

½ red bell pepper, seeded and make ¼-inch rings
1 ½ cups of water
1 ½ tbs. of extra virgin olive oil
1 large yellow potato, make ¼-inch slices
½ yellow onion, make thin slices
2 tbs. of sour cream
4 eggs, beaten
Pepper and salt to taste
¼ cup of cheddar cheese, grated

Nutritional Value (Per Serving):

Calories – 465 | Fat – 10g | Carbohydrate – 36.5g | Fiber – 5g | Protein – 18.5g

Herbal Omelet

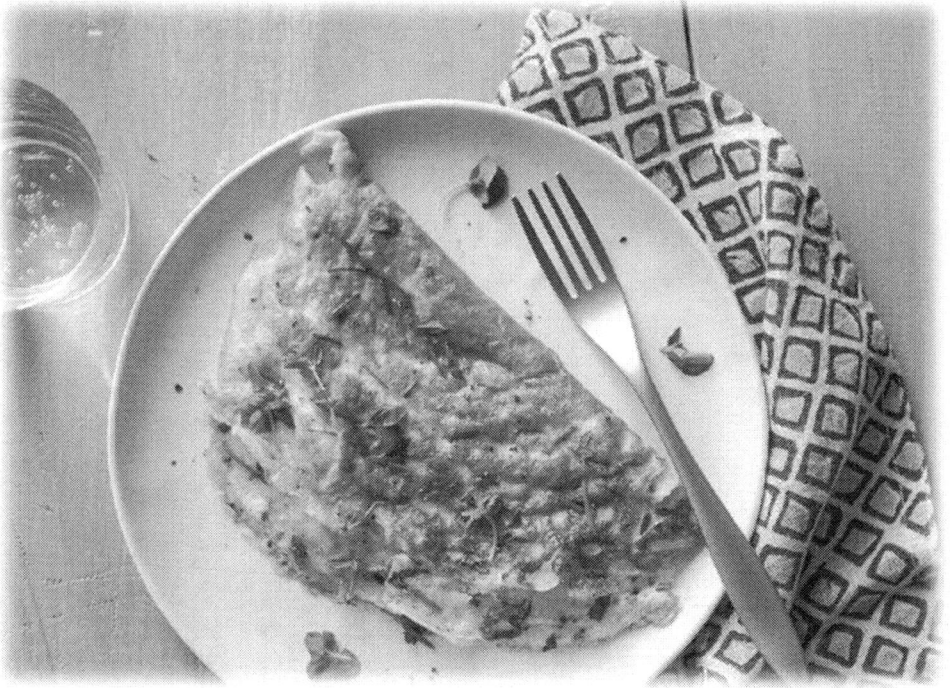

Directions:

- In a bowl of medium size, thoroughly mix the eggs, parsley, thyme, basil, and rosemary. Season it with pepper and salt.
- Switch on your instant pot. Make sure that your kitchen platform is clean and dry.
- Select "Saute" setting from various available options.
- Open the pot and add some butter and egg mixture; cook for 1 minute on each side.
- Add cheese and fold other empty half.
- Cook for 1 minute and serve hot!

Ingredients:

1 ½ tbs. of parsley, finely chopped
1 ½ tbs. of thyme, finely chopped
1 1/2 tbs. of butter
3 eggs, medium
1 ½ tbs. of basil, finely chopped
½ tbs. of shredded cheese, gluten free
1 ½ tbs. of rosemary, finely chopped
A pinch of salt
A pinch of black pepper

Nutritional Value (Per Serving):

Calories – 417 | Fat – 44g | Carbohydrate – 11.5g | Fiber – 0g | Protein – 17g

Oregano Eggplant Morning

Prep Time: 20-25 min. | Serves: 3-4

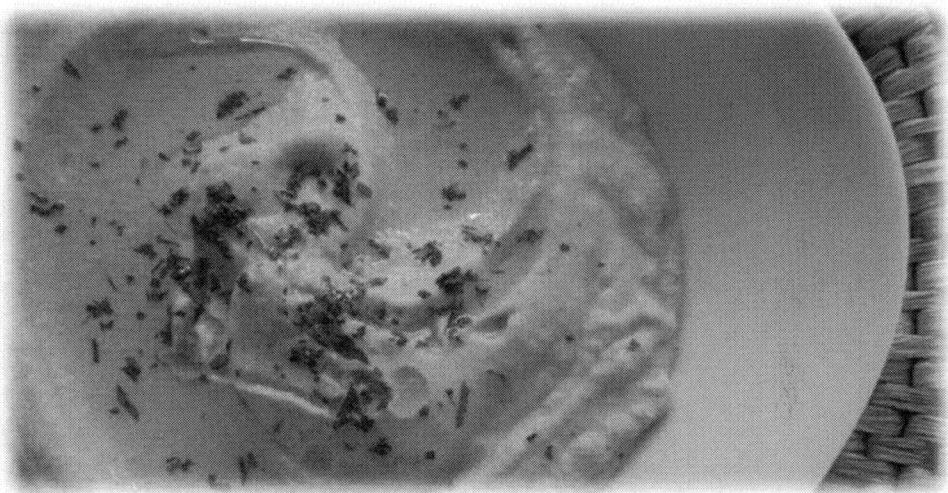

Directions:
- Switch on your instant pot. Make sure that your kitchen platform is clean and dry.
- Select "Saute" setting from various available options.
- Open the pot and add some oil and eggplant cubes; heat for 3-4 minutes to cook well and soften. Stir in between.
- Set aside the eggplant cubes.
- Add in onions and garlic. Saute for 2-3 minutes.
- Add oregano, pepper and salt. Add also cooked eggplant cubes.
- Make sure to lock the lid properly after closing the pot. Also ensure to seal the valve.
- Select "Manual" setting from various available options. Adjust cooking time to 10 minutes.
- Allow the mixture to cook under pressure until the timer reads zero.
- Turn off and press "Cancel" setting.
- Open the pot and transfer the mixture to a blender or food processor.
- Add fronds and pour vinegar. Process until it turns smooth.
- Refrigerate for 1-2 hour.
- Enjoy the eggplant mixture with fresh vegetables, carrots or gluten free crackers.

Ingredients:
- 1 tsp. of oregano, dried
- ½ tsp. of sea salt
- 2 tbs. of olive oil
- 2 large eggplants, cubed
- 2 onions, chopped
- 2 garlic cloves, chopped
- 1 ½ tbs. of balsamic vinegar
- ½ cup of dill fronds, chopped
- ½ tsp. of black pepper

Nutritional Value (Per Serving):
Calories – 176 | Fat – 7g | Carbohydrate – 24g | Fiber – 8.5g | Protein – 3.5g

Cauliflower Cashew Porridge

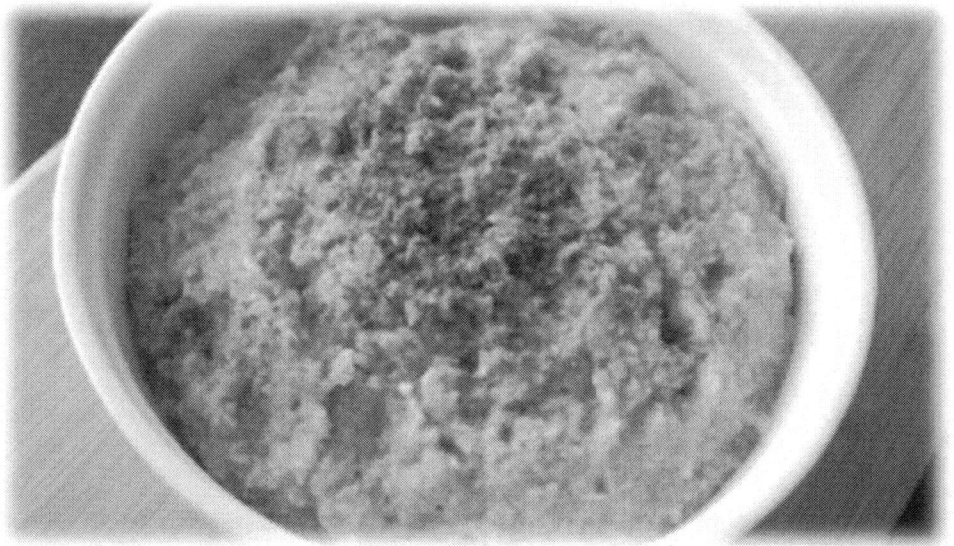

Directions:

- Switch on your instant pot. Make sure that your kitchen platform is clean and dry.
- Select "Saute" setting from various available options.
- Open the pot and add some oil, garlic and leeks; heat for 2 minutes to cook well and soften.
- Add the cauliflower florets inside a blender. Blend for 1 minute.
- Add the stock and cauliflower in the pot and combine well.
- Mix curry powder and cashew nuts. Season it with pepper and salt.
- Make sure to lock the lid properly after closing the pot. Also ensure to seal the valve.
- Select "Manual" setting from various available options. Adjust cooking time to 8 minutes.
- Allow the mixture to cook under pressure until the timer reads zero.
- Turn off and press "Cancel" setting.
- Open the pot and transfer the mixture to a serving bowl.

Ingredients:

2 leeks, minced
1 tsp. of curry powder
1 tbs. of cashew nuts, roughly chopped
1 head cauliflower, make small florets
2 cups of vegetable stock, gluten free
¼ tsp. of olive oil
1 garlic clove, minced
A pinch of salt
A pinch of black pepper

Nutritional Value (Per Serving):

Calories – 492 | Fat – 29g | Carbohydrate – 42g | Fiber – 15g | Protein – 24g

Chapter 2:
Nutritious Lunch Recipes

Mexican Style Soup

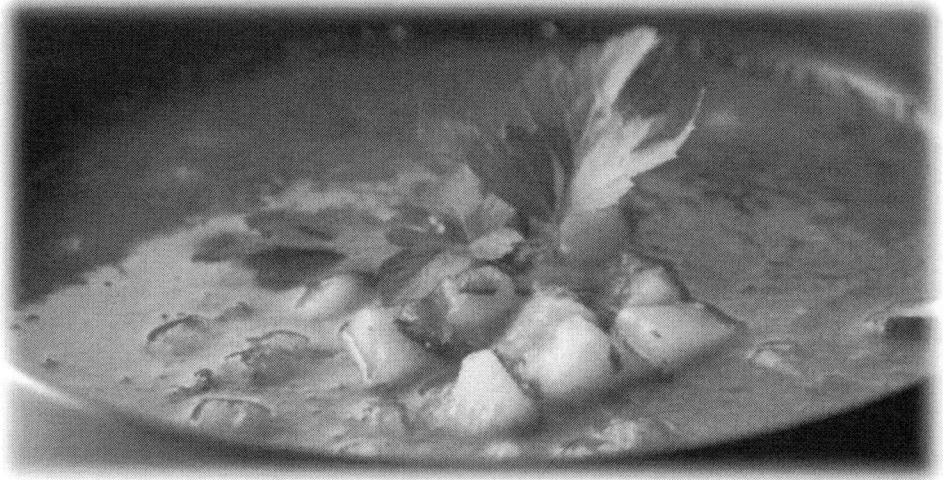

Directions:

- Switch on your instant pot. Make sure that your kitchen platform is clean and dry.
- Select "Saute" setting from various available options.
- Open the pot and add some oil, garlic, jalapeno, and onion; heat for 2 minutes to cook well and soften.
- Add in potatoes, salsa, cumin, oregano and broth.
- Mix all the ingredients.
- Make sure to lock the lid properly after closing the pot. Also ensure to seal the valve.
- Select "Soup/Stew" setting from various available options. Adjust cooking time to 12 minutes.
- Allow the mixture to cook under pressure until the timer reads zero.
- Turn off and press "Cancel" setting.
- Let inside pressure to release naturally; it will take 8-10 minutes for pressure release.
- Open the pot and transfer the mixture to a blender.
- Make a smooth puree.
- Add yeast and pepper; mix and serve hot!

Ingredients:

1 tsp. of cumin
¼ tsp. of oregano
½ cup of salsa to your taste (gluten-free)
⅛ cup of jalapeno peppers, seeded
1 onion, diced
½ cup of nutritional yeast
4 cups of potatoes, make small pieces
4 cups of veggie broth, gluten free
4 diced garlic cloves
Black pepper as needed

Nutritional Value (Per Serving):

Calories – 194 | Fat – 0.5g | Carbohydrate – 27.5g | Fiber – 4g | Protein – 10.5g

Chicken Bean Tortilla

Prep Time: 10-15 min. | Serves: 4-5

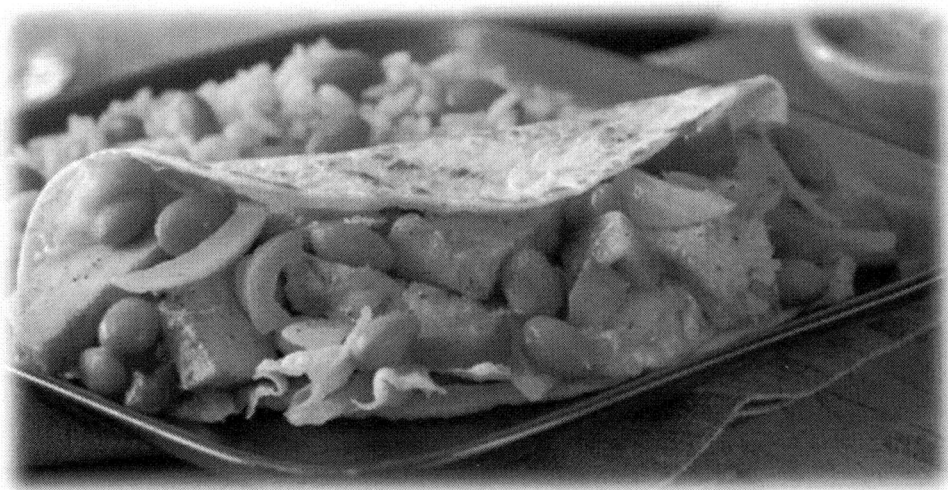

Directions:

- Switch on your instant pot. Make sure that your kitchen platform is clean and dry.
- Select "Saute" setting from various available options.
- Open the pot and add some oil, chicken, garlic and onions; heat for 2 minutes to cook well and soften.
- Add tomatoes, cinnamon, peppers, and raisins.
- Make sure to lock the lid properly after closing the pot. Also ensure to seal the valve.
- Select "Manual" setting from various available options. Adjust cooking time to 5 minutes.
- Allow the mixture to cook under pressure until the timer reads zero.
- Turn off and press "Cancel" setting.
- Add the mixture over corn tortillas; add bean and pepper.
- Wrap and serve!

Ingredients:

2 tsp. of garlic, minced
1 pound of chicken breasts, skinless and boneless
1 can of tomatoes, diced
1 tbs. of olive oil
2 white onions, chopped
1 mild chili pepper, chopped
½ cup of raisins
1 cinnamon stick
1 sweet red peppers, chopped
1 sweet red peppers, make strips
8 corn tortillas, gluten free
Beans and red pepper flakes as needed

Nutritional Value (Per Serving):
Calories – 328 | Fat – 10.5g | Carbohydrate – 22g | Fiber – 2g | Protein – 21g

Beef Patties with Vegetables

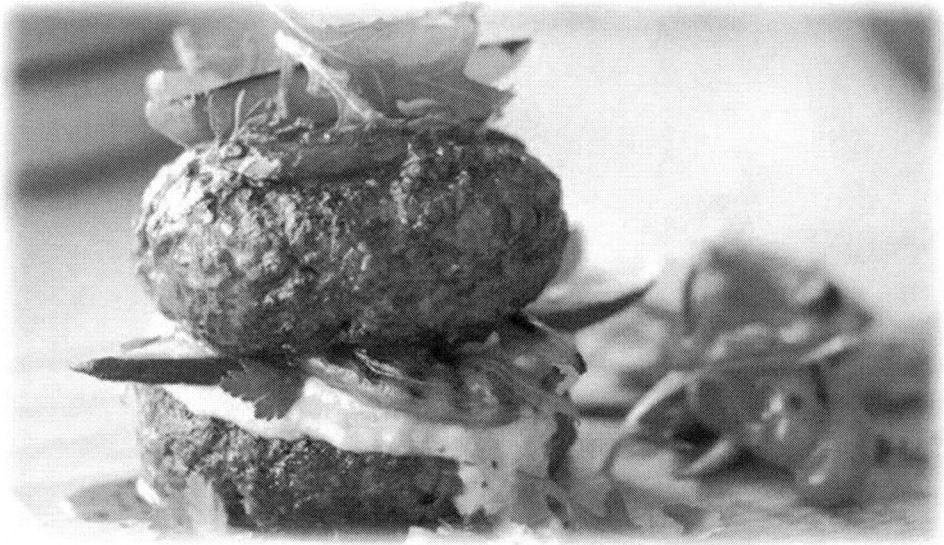

Directions:

- In a bowl of medium size, thoroughly mix beef, Worcestershire sauce, salt, pepper and garlic powder.
- Form into 4 balls; flatten with plate.
- Top 2 patties with 1 slice each of Gouda and top with leftover patties; seal edges.
- Switch on your instant pot. Make sure that your kitchen platform is clean and dry.
- Pour the water in the pot. Arrange a trivet inside and add the patties over the trivet.
- Make sure to lock the lid properly after closing the pot. Also ensure to seal the valve.
- Select "Manual" setting from various available options. Adjust cooking time to 5 minutes.
- Allow the mixture to cook under pressure until the timer reads zero.
- Turn off and press "Cancel" setting.
- Open the pot.
- Serve the patties with additional toppings as desired.
- You can enjoy the patties with your favorite salads also.

Ingredients:

1 pound of lean beef, ground
2 slices of smoked Gouda cheese
1 cup of water
1 tbs. of Worcestershire sauce
Pepper and salt to taste
Garlic powder as needed
Topping choices: tomato, lettuce, pickles, sprouts, and/or avocados

Nutritional Value (Per Serving):

Calories – 515 | Fat – 32.5g | Carbohydrate – 2g | Fiber – 1g | Protein – 52g

Ginger Squash Soup

Prep Time: 15-20 min. | Serves: 2-3

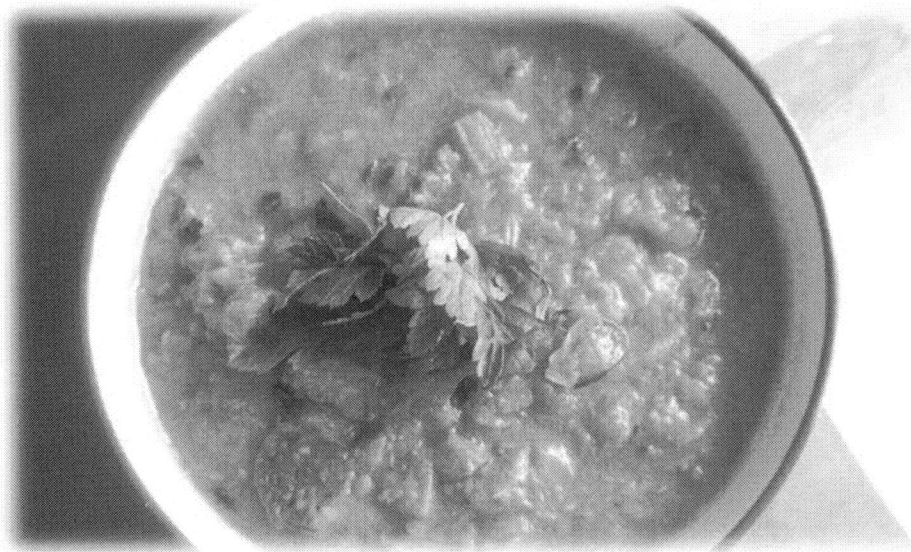

Directions:

- Switch on your instant pot. Make sure that your kitchen platform is clean and dry.
- Select "Saute" setting from various available options.
- Open the pot and add some salt, ginger, coconut oil, garlic, and onion; heat for 2 minutes to cook well and soften.
- Add the remaining ingredients and stir well.
- Make sure to lock the lid properly after closing the pot. Also ensure to seal the valve.
- Select "Manual" setting from various available options. Adjust cooking time to 10 minutes.
- Allow the mixture to cook under pressure until the timer reads zero.
- Turn off and press "Cancel" setting.
- Open the pot.
- Add the mixture to a food processor, and blend until it's smooth. Serve hot!

Ingredients:

2 cups of sweet potatoes, peeled and make cubes
½ tsp. of nutmeg
3 cups of vegetable broth, gluten-free
2 cups of peeled butternut squash, de-seeded, chopped
1 tsp. of tarragon
1 tsp. of cinnamon
1 onion, chopped
½ tsp. of turmeric
1-inch ginger piece, peeled
1 ½ tsp. of curry powder
2 garlic cloves, crushed
1 tsp. of salt
2 tbs. of coconut oil

Nutritional Value (Per Serving):

Calories – 292 | Fat – 11g | Carbohydrate – 48g | Fiber – 11g | Protein – 3.5g

Bean Vegetable Lunch Meal

Prep Time: 20-25 min. | Serves: 6-8

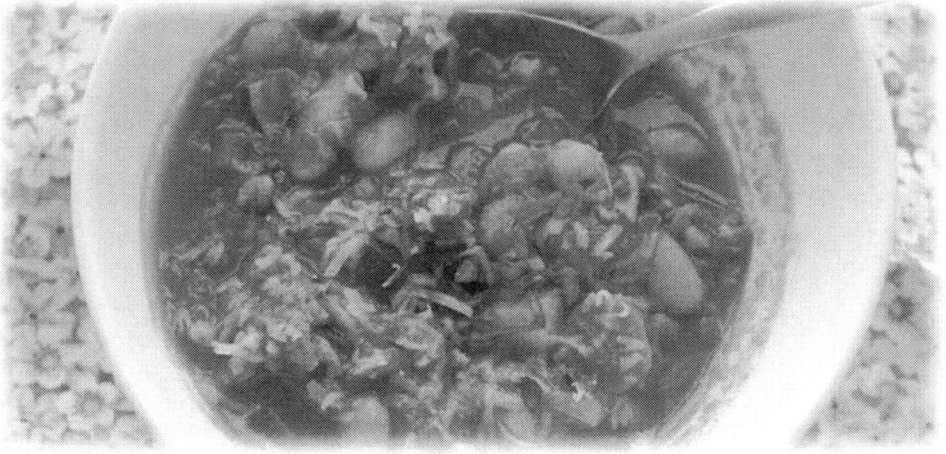

Directions:

- Switch on your instant pot. Make sure that your kitchen platform is clean and dry.
- Select "Saute" setting from various available options.
- Open the pot and add some oil, garlic, and onion; heat for 2-3 minutes to cook well and soften.
- Add 1 pack of veggie round and brown it.
- Add chili powder, bell pepper, cumin, oregano, salt and black pepper; combine well.
- Add beans, tomatoes and water; stir well.
- Make sure to lock the lid properly after closing the pot. Also ensure to seal the valve.
- Select "Manual" setting from various available options. Adjust cooking time to 20 minutes.
- Allow the mixture to cook under pressure until the timer reads zero.
- Turn off and press "Cancel" setting. Naturally release pressure.
- Open the pot and transfer the mixture to a serving bowl.
- Serve hot!

Ingredients:

1 tsp. of garlic, minced
1 (12 oz.) pack of veggie ground round, gluten-free
1 diced red bell pepper
2 tsp. of cumin
1 tbs. of chili powder
2 tbs. of olive oil
2 yellow onions, chopped
1 tsp. of oregano
Pepper and salt to taste
14 ounces of Roma tomatoes, chopped
8 ounces of pinto beans, soaked
8 ounces of kidney beans, soaked
4 cups of water

Nutritional Value (Per Serving):

Calories – 255 | Fat – 9g | Carbohydrate – 28g | Fiber – 10g | Protein – 17g

Garlic Ham Soup

Prep Time: 50-60 min. | Serves: 5-6

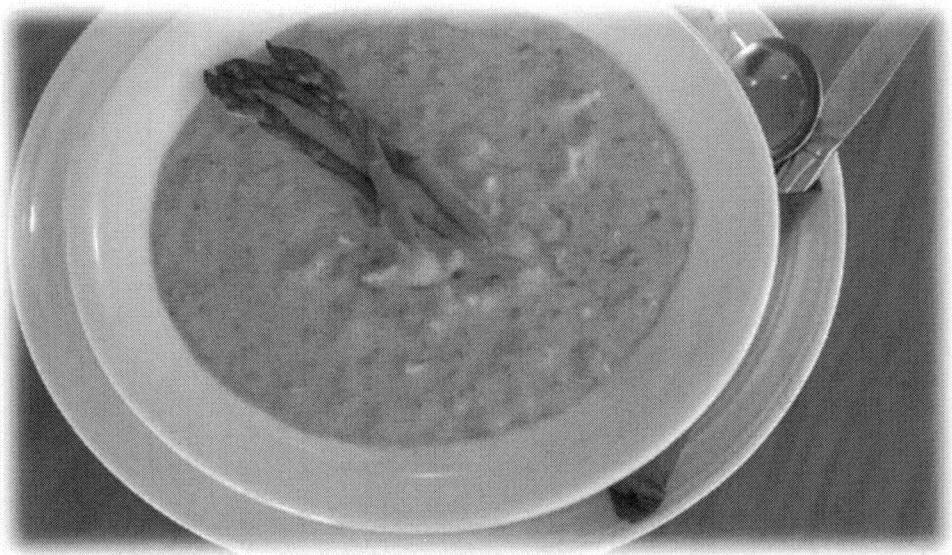

Directions:
- Switch on your instant pot. Make sure that your kitchen platform is clean and dry.
- Select "Saute" setting from various available options.
- Open the pot and add some oil and onions; heat for 2 minutes to cook well and soften.
- Add in garlic and ham; combine and pour in the broth.
- Simmer the mix for a few minutes.
- Add asparagus and thyme; stir well.
- Make sure to lock the lid properly after closing the pot. Also ensure to seal the valve.
- Select "Manual" setting from various available options. Adjust cooking time to 55 minutes.
- Allow the mixture to cook under pressure until the timer reads zero.
- Turn off and press "Cancel" setting.
- Open the pot.
- Puree in blender until the soup becomes smooth.
- Add pepper and salt; mix and serve!

Ingredients:
1 onion, diced
2 pounds of split asparagus
5 pressed garlic cloves
1 cup of ham, diced
4 cups of chicken broth, gluten free
½ tsp. of thyme, dried
Salt to taste

Nutritional Value (Per Serving):
Calories – 283 | Fat – 16g | Carbohydrate – 18g | Fiber – 2.5g | Protein – 13g

Chicken Bean Tortilla Soup

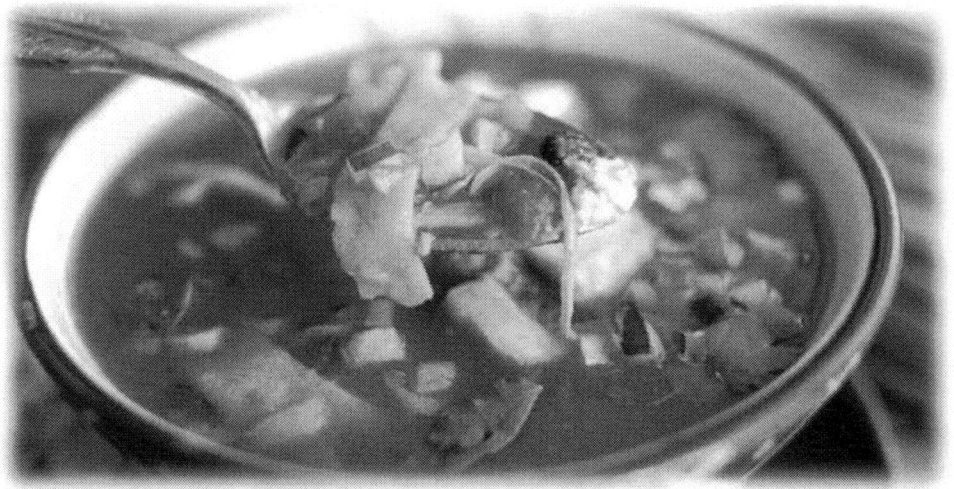

Directions:

- Switch on your instant pot. Make sure that your kitchen platform is clean and dry.
- Select "Saute" setting from various available options.
- Open the pot and add some oil and onions; heat for 2 minutes to cook well and soften.
- Add tortilla pieces, cilantro, and garlic, and stir well.
- Cook for 1 minute; in the pot, add beans, corn, spices, broth, and chicken. Stir well.
- Make sure to lock the lid properly after closing the pot. Also ensure to seal the valve.
- Select "Soup" setting from various available options. Adjust cooking time to 4 minutes.
- Allow the mixture to cook under pressure until the timer reads zero.
- Turn off and press "Cancel" setting.
- Open the pot and transfer the mixture to a serving bowl.
- Using two forks, shred the chicken, and place it back.
- Stir well and serve hot!

Ingredients:

1 tbs. of olive oil
3 chicken breasts
1 onion, chopped
1 bay leaf
2 minced garlic cloves
¼ tsp. of cayenne pepper
2 gluten-free corn tortillas, chopped
1 tsp. of cumin
2 tbs. of cilantro
1 cup of corn, frozen
2 tsp. of chili powder
1 large tomato, chopped
3 cups of gluten-free chicken broth
2 cups of black beans

Nutritional Value (Per Serving):

Calories – 313 | Fat – 8g | Carbohydrate – 23g | Fiber – 3g | Protein – 34g

Tangy Chicken Lentil Soup

Prep Time: 35-40 min. | Serves: 4-5

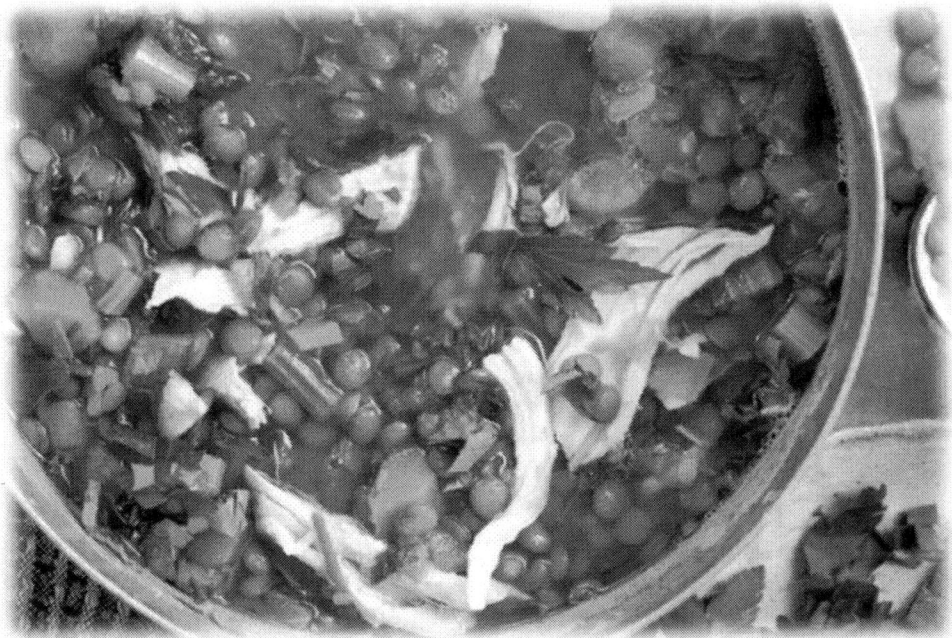

Directions:
- Switch on your instant pot. Make sure that your kitchen platform is clean and dry.
- Open the lid and gradually add all the above mentioned ingredients in the pot.
- Make sure to lock the lid properly after closing the pot. Also ensure to seal the valve.
- Select "Soup" setting from various available options. Adjust cooking time to 30 minutes.
- Allow the mixture to cook under pressure until the timer reads zero.
- Turn off and press "Cancel" setting.
- Open the pot and transfer the mixture to a serving bowl.
- Using two forks, shred the chicken, and place it back.
- Stir well and serve hot!

Ingredients:
1 tbs. of gluten-free bouillon
2 cups of uncooked lentils
¼ tsp. of salt
1 ½ boneless chicken thighs, trimmed
½ tsp. of cumin
½ onion, chopped
½ tsp. of garlic powder
¼ tsp. of paprika
3 ½ cups of water
A pinch of oregano
1 scallion, chopped
½ tomato, chopped
1/8 cup of cilantro
1 ½ garlic cloves, chopped

Nutritional Value (Per Serving):
Calories – 202 | Fat – 1g | Carbohydrate – 42.5g | Fiber – 15.5g | Protein – 17g

Healthy Vegetable Soup

Prep Time: 12-15 min. | Serves: 4-5

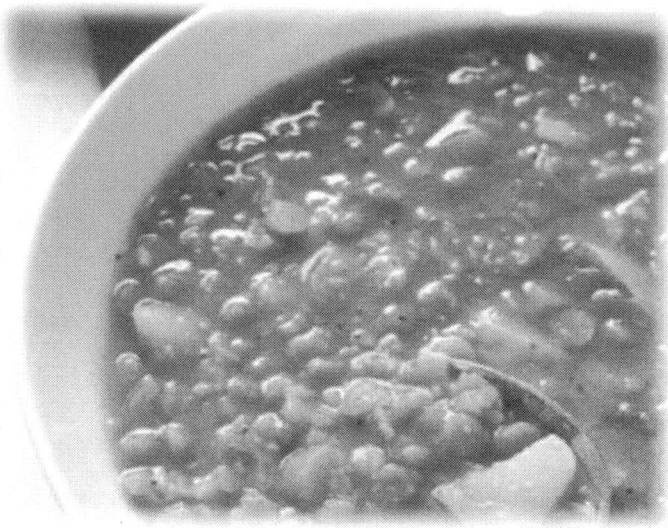

Directions:
- Switch on your instant pot. Make sure that your kitchen platform is clean and dry.
- Select "Saute" setting from various available options.
- Open the pot and add some oil and leek; heat for 1 minute to cook well and soften.
- Add garlic; cook for another 1 minute.
- Press "cancel"; in the pot, add in broth, parsnips, celery root, lentils, carrots, and herbs.
- Make sure to lock the lid properly after closing the pot. Also ensure to seal the valve.
- Select "Soup/stew" setting from various available options. Adjust cooking time to 7 minutes.
- Allow the mixture to cook under pressure until the timer reads zero.
- Turn off and press "Cancel" setting.
- Open the pot and add in the peas, stir well.
- Close the lid and just let the mixture sit for 2-3 minutes.
- Add in some salt, pepper, and lemon juice.
- Serve the soup hot!

Ingredients:
1 sprig rosemary
½ cup of peas, frozen
½ cup of green lentils
1 ½ cups of broth
1 cup of sliced leek
1 cup of parsnip, diced
1 cup of carrot, diced
3 cups of celery root, diced
2 bay leaves
1 sprig thyme
A few drops of lemon juice
Pepper and salt to taste

Nutritional Value (Per Serving):
Calories – 98 | Fat – 0g | Carbohydrate – 22.5g | Fiber – 5g | Protein – 3.5g

Chicken Potato Stew

Prep Time: 35-40 min. | Serves: 6-7

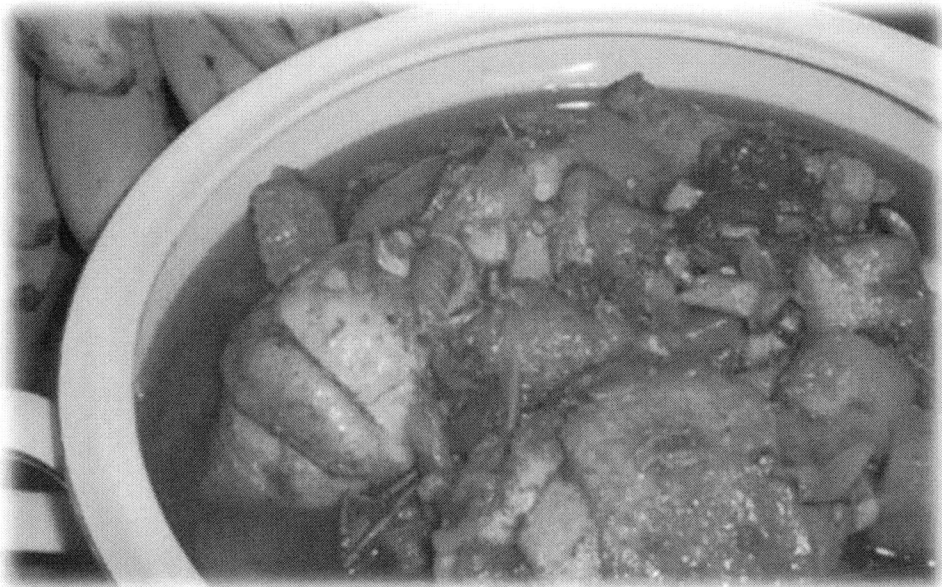

Directions:

- Switch on your instant pot. Make sure that your kitchen platform is clean and dry.
- Open the lid and gradually add all the above mentioned ingredients in the pot.
- Make sure to lock the lid properly after closing the pot. Also ensure to seal the valve.
- Select "Chicken/Meat" setting from various available options. Adjust cooking time to 30 minutes.
- Allow the mixture to cook under pressure until the timer reads zero.
- Turn off and press "Cancel" setting.
- Open the pot and transfer the mixture to a serving bowl.
- Season as required before serving.

Ingredients:

½ cup of chicken broth
4 pounds of chicken breasts
3 cups of tomatoes, make small pieces
2 bay leaves
4 large potatoes, peeled and chopped
1 sliced onion
Pepper and salt to taste

Nutritional Value (Per Serving):

Calories – 291 | Fat – 8.5g | Carbohydrate – 13g | Fiber – 1g | Protein – 34.5g

Chapter 3:
Wholesome Dinners

Shrimp Garlic Rice

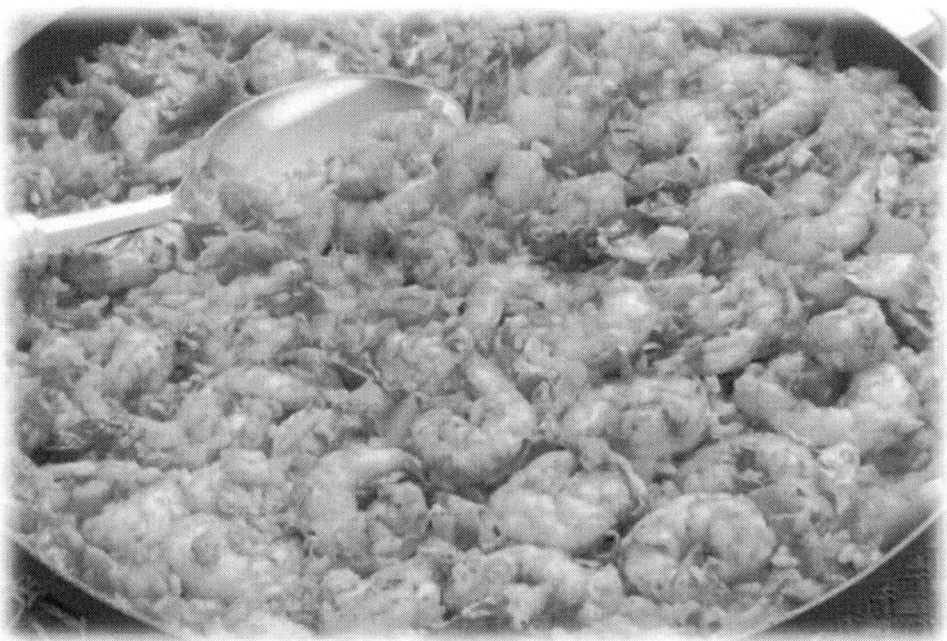

Directions:
- Switch on your instant pot. Make sure that your kitchen platform is clean and dry.
- Open the lid and gradually add the above mentioned ingredients in the pot. Add shrimp last.
- Make sure to lock the lid properly after closing the pot. Also ensure to seal the valve.
- Select "Manual" setting from various available options. Adjust cooking time to 5 minutes.
- Allow the mixture to cook under pressure until the timer reads zero.
- Turn off and press "Cancel" setting.
- Open the pot and transfer the mixture to a serving bowl.
- Serve hot!

Ingredients:
1 cup of jasmine rice, gluten free
1 1/2 cups of water
1/4 cup of chopped parsley
Juice of 1 lemon
1 pound of shrimp
4 minced garlic cloves
1/4 cup of butter
A pinch of saffron
1 tsp. of sea salt
A pinch of red pepper
1/4 tsp. of black pepper

Nutritional Value (Per Serving):
Calories – 266 | Fat – 13g | Carbohydrate – 14g | Fiber – 0g | Protein – 24g

Vegetarian Chili Dinner

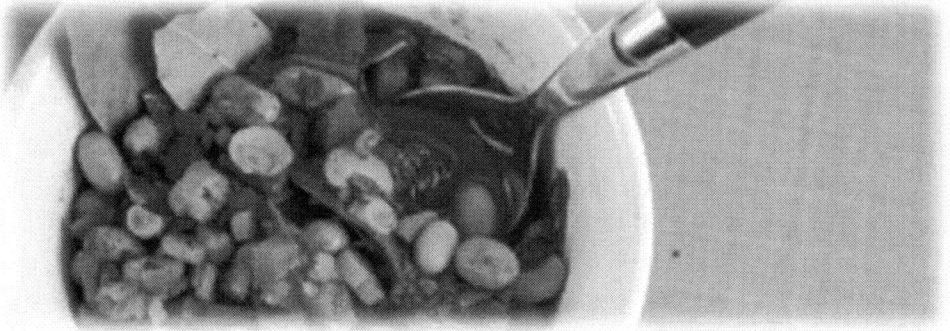

Directions:

- Cut collard greens lengthwise and remove inner ribs; divide them crosswise to make strips about 6mm wide.
- Switch on your instant pot. Make sure that your kitchen platform is clean and dry.
- Select "Saute" setting from various available options.
- Open the pot and add oil, garlic and onions; heat for 2 minutes to cook well and soften.
- Add celery and carrots, cook for 4-5 minutes.
- Add cumin, greens, chili powder, coriander, oregano, cinnamon and jalapeno; cook for 1 minute.
- Add water, black-eyed peas, bay leaves, tomato sauce, tomatoes, and broth.
- Make sure to lock the lid properly after closing the pot. Also ensure to seal the valve.
- Select "Manual" setting from various available options. Adjust cooking time to 10 minutes.
- Allow the mixture to cook under pressure until the timer reads zero.
- Turn off and press "Cancel" setting.
- Open the pot and transfer the mixture to a serving bowl.
- Remove bay leaves before serving.

Ingredients:

1 cup of diced onion
2 cups of celery, chopped
2 cups of carrots, chopped
4 large collard green leaves
1 tsp. of olive oil
2 tsp. of minced garlic
1 tsp. of ground cumin
2 tbs. of chili powder
½ tsp. of ground coriander
1 tbs. of oregano
1 tsp. of cinnamon
1 jalapeno, seeded and diced
1 cup of water
2 cups of black-eyed peas, dried
2 bay leaves
8 ounces of tomato sauce, homemade
28 ounces of diced tomatoes
2 cups of vegetable broth, low-sodium, gluten free
Green onion, chopped for garnish
Sea salt to taste

Nutritional Value (Per Serving):

Calories – 192 | Fat – 1.5g | Carbohydrate – 41g | Fiber – 11g | Protein – 6g

Chicken Onion Adobo

Prep Time: 7 hours 15-20 min. | Serves: 4

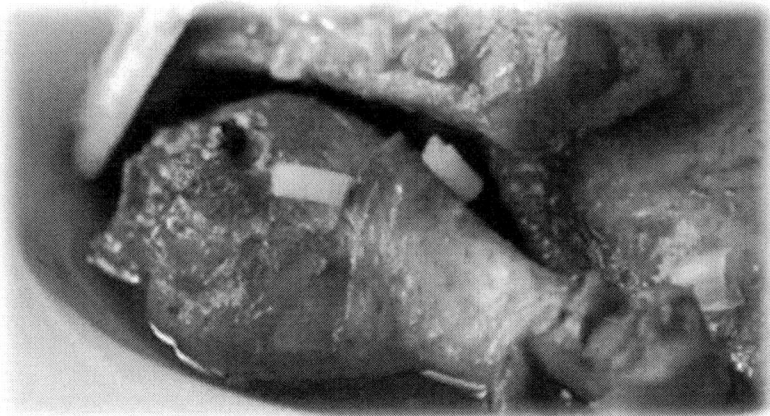

Directions:
- In a bowl of medium size, thoroughly mix the soy sauces, fish sauce, sugar, and vinegar.
- Switch on your instant pot. Make sure that your kitchen platform is clean and dry.
- Select "Saute" setting from various available options.
- Open the pot and add the oil and chicken; heat for 2 minutes to cook well and soften.
- Then remove it from the pot, and set to one side.
- Add the onion, some oil and garlic and cook for a few minutes.
- Mix the bay leaves, pepper, and chili. Cook for 30-40 seconds.
- Mix the bowl mixture, chicken and stir, de-glazing the pot as you do.
- Make sure to lock the lid properly after closing the pot. Also ensure to seal the valve.
- Select "Manual" setting from various available options. Adjust cooking time to 9 minutes.
- Allow the mixture to cook under pressure until the timer reads zero.
- Turn off and press "Cancel" setting. Naturally release pressure.
- Open the pot and transfer the mixture in serving bowl.
- Sprinkle the onions on top and serve.

Ingredients:
1/4 cup soy sauce, gluten free
4 dried bay leaves
2 pounds chicken
2 green onions, chopped
1 tbs. oil
1/2 cup soy sauce, gluten free
1 dried red chili
1 tbs. fish sauce
1 onion, sliced
1/4 cup vinegar
1 tsp. black pepper
1 tbs. sugar
10 garlic cloves, crushed

Nutritional Value (Per Serving):
Calories – 534 | Fat – 34g | Carbohydrate – 42g | Fiber – 6g | Protein – 44.5g

Chicken Tomatino Feast

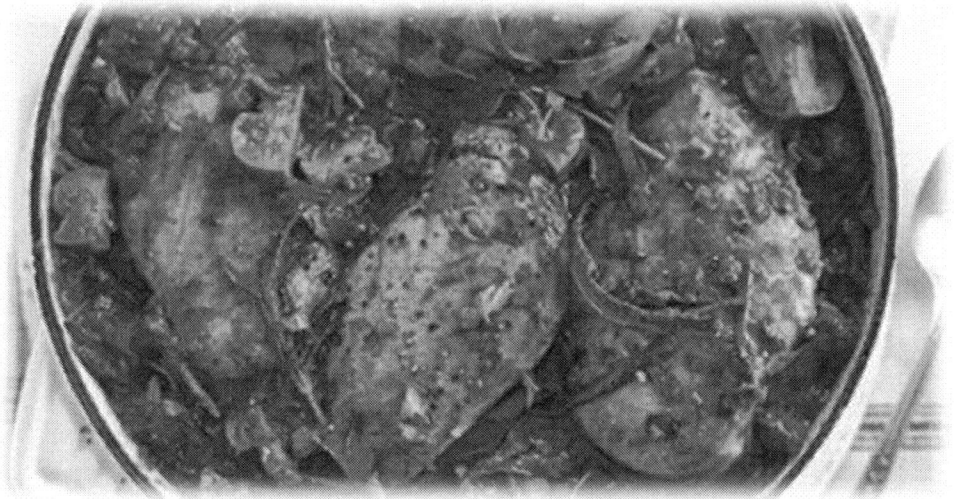

Directions:

- Season chicken with pepper and salt.
- Switch on your instant pot. Make sure that your kitchen platform is clean and dry.
- Select "Saute" setting from various available options.
- Open the pot and add oil and chicken; heat to brown evenly and set aside.
- Add onion to pot and sauté for 4-5 minutes; add garlic, red pepper flakes and oregano.
- Add bay leaf, tomatoes and broth; return chicken to pot.
- Make sure to lock the lid properly after closing the pot. Also ensure to seal the valve.
- Select "Manual" setting from various available options. Adjust cooking time to 10 minutes.
- Allow the mixture to cook under pressure until the timer reads zero.
- Turn off and press "Cancel" setting.
- Open the pot and add green peppers.
- Close the lid and cook for 2 more minutes. Quick release pressure and remove bay leaf.
- Serve along with cooked rice.

Ingredients:

2 tbs. of olive oil
2 pounds of chicken thighs, boneless, skinless
1 white onion, minced
1 tsp. of garlic, minced
¼ tsp. of red pepper flakes
1 tsp. of oregano
1 bay leaf
¼ cup of chicken broth, gluten free
28 ounces of diced tomatoes
2 green bell peppers, diced
Pepper and salt to taste

Nutritional Value (Per Serving):

Calories – 236 | Fat – 5g | Carbohydrate – 9.5g | Fiber – 2.5g | Protein – 32g

Beef Chili Stew

Prep Time: 1 hours 5-10 min. | Serves: 3

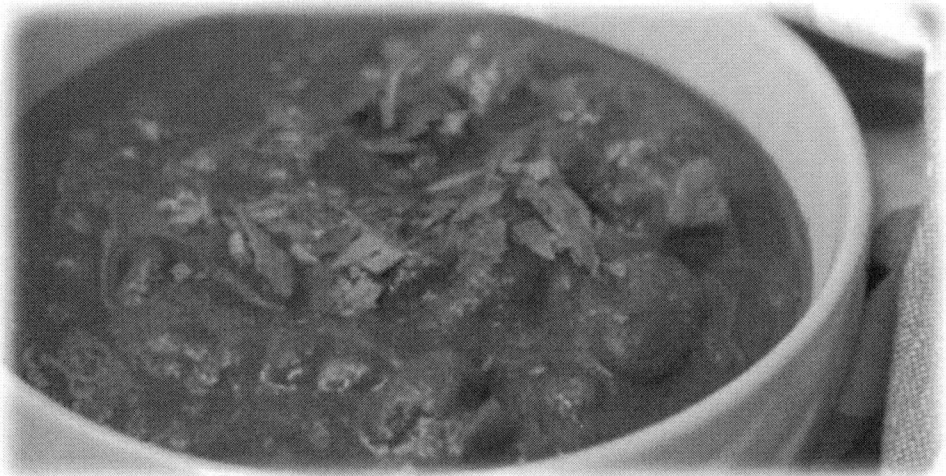

Directions:

- In a bowl of medium size, thoroughly mix the chili powder, beef, and salt.
- Switch on your instant pot. Make sure that your kitchen platform is clean and dry.
- Select "Saute" setting from various available options.
- Open the pot and add some butter and onions; heat for 2 minutes to cook well and soften.
- Add the garlic and tomato paste. Cook for 20-30 seconds. Now add the beef and stir.
- Add fish sauce, stock, and salsa; combine well.
- Make sure to lock the lid properly after closing the pot. Also ensure to seal the valve.
- Select "Meat" setting from various available options. Adjust cooking time to 35 minutes.
- Allow the mixture to cook under pressure until the timer reads zero.
- Turn off and press "Cancel" setting.
- Open the pot and transfer the mixture to a serving bowl.
- Season the stew and serve hot!

Ingredients:

1/4 tsp. of fish sauce
3/4 tsp. of salt
1/4 cup of gluten-free bone broth
1 tbs. of butter
1/4 cup of tomato salsa
1 1/4 pounds of beef chuck roast, make cubes
A pinch of black pepper
1/2 tbs. of chili powder
1 onion, chopped
1/2 tbs. of tomato paste
3 garlic cloves, crushed

Nutritional Value (Per Serving):

Calories – 512 | Fat – 36g | Carbohydrate – 8g | Fiber – 1g | Protein – 37.5g

Instant Black Bean Pork Ribs

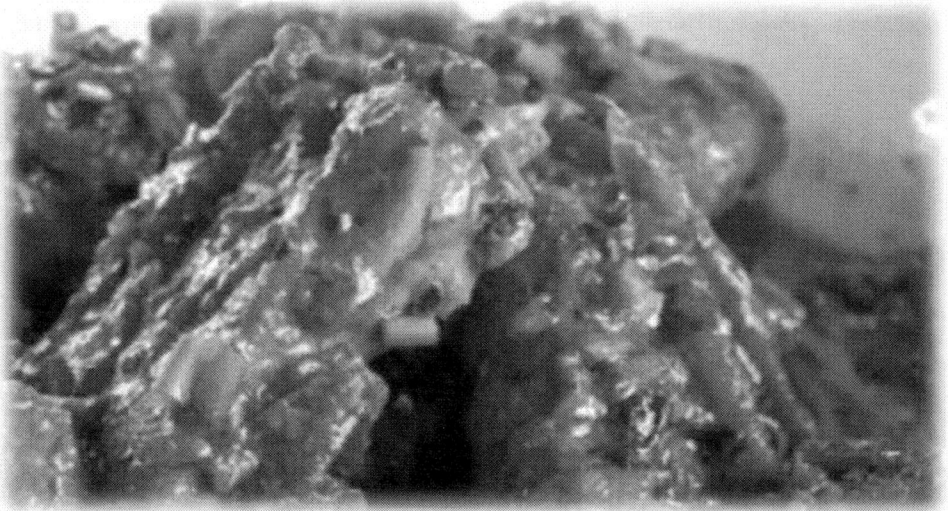

Directions:

- In a bowl of medium size, thoroughly mix all the ingredients apart from the spare ribs, water, and cornstarch.
- Now add spare ribs, and coat well. Marinade at room temperature for 30-45 minutes.
- Add cornstarch, and stir well.
- Switch on your instant pot. Make sure that your kitchen platform is clean and dry.
- Open the lid and gradually add water, ribs and bowl mixture in the pot.
- Make sure to lock the lid properly after closing the pot. Also ensure to seal the valve.
- Select "Meat" setting from various available options. Adjust cooking time to 15 minutes.
- Allow the mixture to cook under pressure until the timer reads zero.
- Turn off and press "Cancel" setting.
- Open the pot and transfer the mixture to a serving bowl.
- Serve hot!

Ingredients:

1 tsp. of chili
1 tsp. of garlic sauce
1 tbs. of sesame oil
1/4 cup of crushed garlic
3 tbs. of black beans
1 1/2 tbs. of dry sherry
2 1/2 pounds of pork spare ribs
1/2 cup of chopped green onions
2 tsp. of brown sugar
1 1/2 tbs. of soy sauce, gluten free
2 tsp. of cornstarch
1 tsp. of black pepper
1 cup of water
1 1/2 tsp. of salt

Nutritional Value (Per Serving):

Calories – 123 | Fat – 8g | Carbohydrate – 8g | Fiber – 1g | Protein – 3g

Seasoned Steak

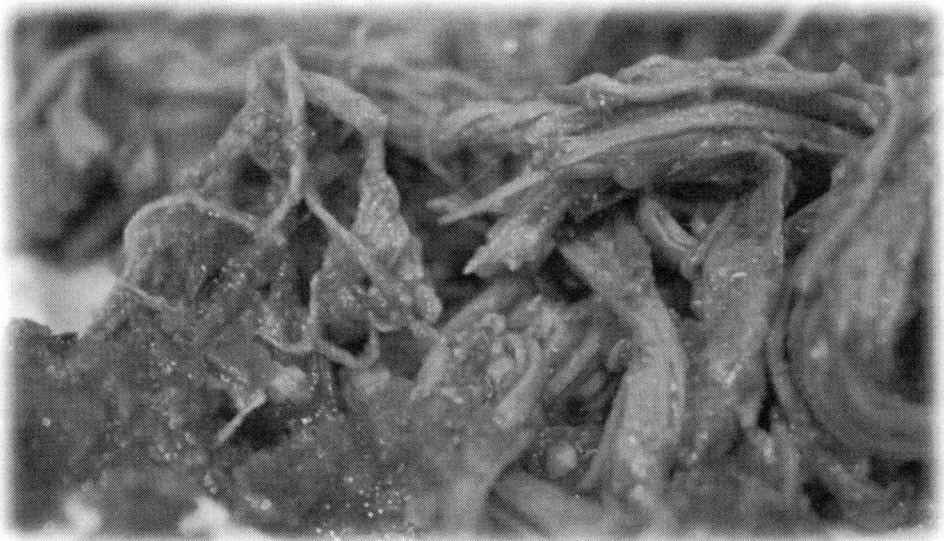

Directions:

- Season steak with salt.
- Switch on your instant pot. Make sure that your kitchen platform is clean and dry.
- Select "Saute" setting from various available options.
- Open the pot and add steak, broth, garlic and onion; heat the mixture and boil it.
- Make sure to lock the lid properly after closing the pot. Also ensure to seal the valve.
- Select "Meat" setting from various available options. Adjust cooking time to 20 minutes.
- Allow the mixture to cook under pressure until the timer reads zero.
- Turn off and press "Cancel" setting.
- Open the pot and transfer the mixture to a serving bowl.
- Remove steak; shred and season with your favorite seasonings.

Ingredients:

2 pounds of flank steak
1 cup of chicken broth, low-sodium, gluten free
2 tsp. of garlic, minced
A dash of sea salt
1 large of onion, quartered
Black pepper to taste

Nutritional Value (Per Serving):
Calories – 445 | Fat – 21g | Carbohydrate – 2g | Fiber – 0g | Protein – 52g

Parmesan Spaghetti Pasta

Prep Time: 8-10 min. | Serves: 4

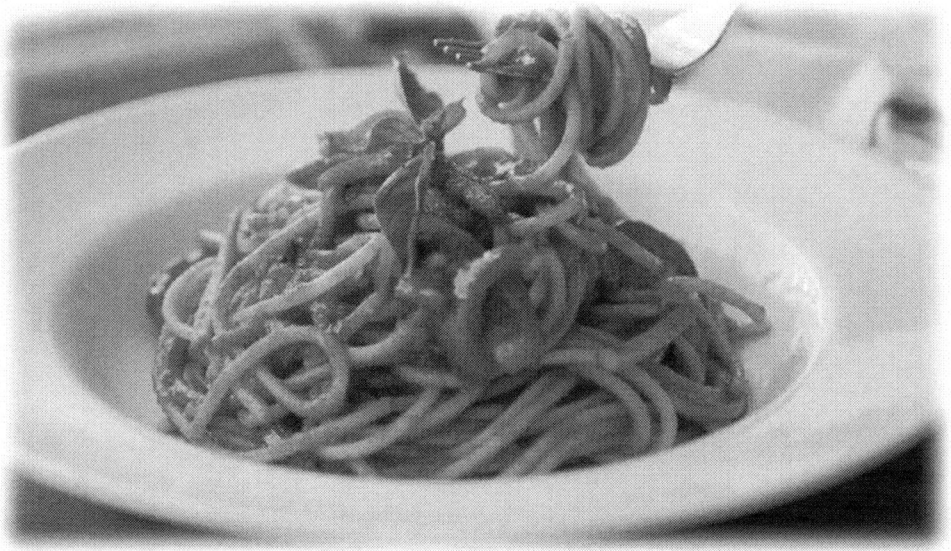

Directions:

- Cut squash and remove the seeds.
- Switch on your instant pot. Make sure that your kitchen platform is clean and dry.
- Open the lid and gradually add the squash and one cup of water in the pot.
- Make sure to lock the lid properly after closing the pot. Also ensure to seal the valve.
- Select "Manual" setting from various available options. Adjust cooking time to 5 minutes.
- Allow the mixture to cook under pressure until the timer reads zero.
- Turn off and press "Cancel" setting.
- Cool down the squash for 5 minutes. Using 2 forks, shred the squash to make it look like spaghetti.
- Select "Saute" setting from various available options.
- Open the pot and add oil and garlic; heat for 2 minutes to cook well and soften.
- Add red pepper and cook for 2-3 seconds.
- Add the squash and season. Add cheese and parsley.
- Combine the mixture well and serve hot!

Ingredients:

1 spaghetti squash
1/4 cup of minced parsley
1/4 cup of olive oil
Salt to taste
6 cloves garlic, crushed
1 cup of Parmesan cheese, grated
1/2 tsp. of red pepper flakes

Nutritional Value (Per Serving):

Calories – 544 | Fat – 38g | Carbohydrate – 6g | Fiber – 0g | Protein – 38g

Spiced Instant Chicken

Prep Time: 30-40 min. | Serves: 4

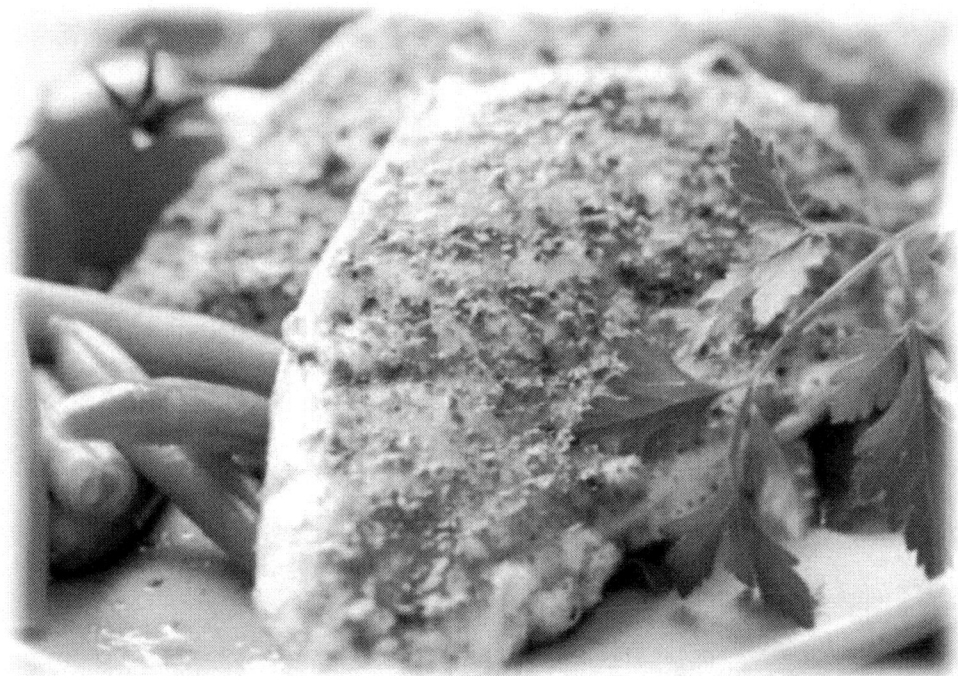

Directions:
- In a bowl of medium size, thoroughly mix all the ingredients and refrigerate overnight.
- Switch on your instant pot. Make sure that your kitchen platform is clean and dry.
- Open the lid and gradually add the mixture in the pot.
- Make sure to lock the lid properly after closing the pot. Also ensure to seal the valve.
- Select "Chicken/Meat" setting from various available options. Adjust cooking time to 25 minutes.
- Allow the mixture to cook under pressure until the timer reads zero.
- Turn off and press "Cancel" setting. Naturally release pressure.
- Open the pot and transfer the mixture to a serving bowl.
- Garnish with green onion and serve.

Ingredients:
½ tsp. of ginger, ground
½ tsp. of cinnamon
4 boneless and skinless chicken breasts
1 tsp. of garlic, minced
2 tsp. of olive oil
½ tsp. of black pepper
1 tsp. of cumin
1 green onion, chopped to garnish

Nutritional Value (Per Serving):
Calories – 65 | Fat – 3g | Carbohydrate – 7g | Fiber – 4g | Protein – 1.5g

Cooked Ham with Wholesome Veggies

Prep Time: 35-40 min. | Serves: 3-4

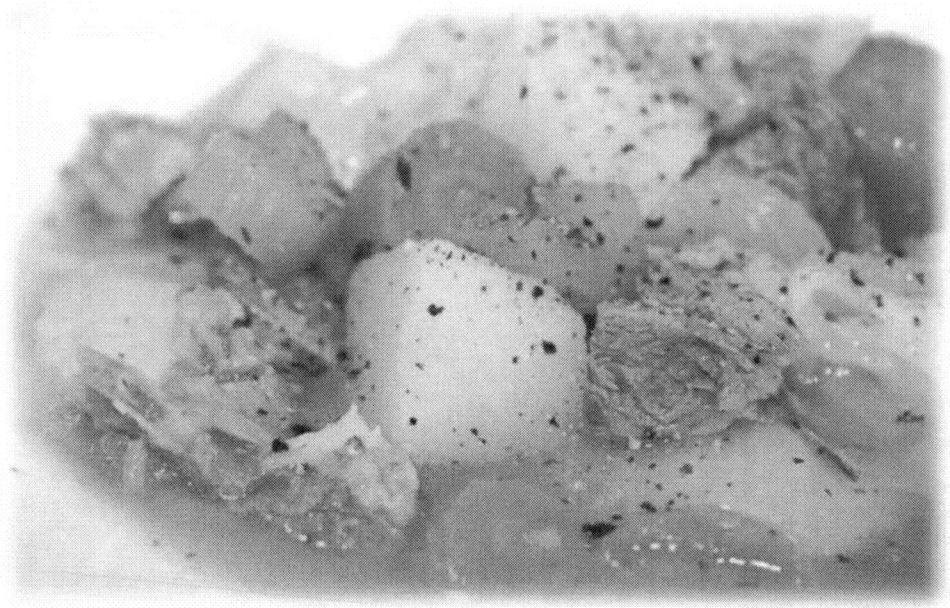

Directions:

- Switch on your instant pot. Make sure that your kitchen platform is clean and dry.
- Open the lid and gradually add all the above mentioned ingredients in the pot. Stir gently.
- Make sure to lock the lid properly after closing the pot. Also ensure to seal the valve.
- Select "Chicken/Meat" setting from various available options. Adjust cooking time to 20 minutes.
- Allow the mixture to cook under pressure until the timer reads zero.
- Turn off and press "Cancel" setting. Naturally release pressure.
- Open the pot and transfer the mixture to a serving bowl.
- Serve hot!

Ingredients:

1 tsp. of chili powder
1 potato, large piece and chopped
1 onion, minced
1 pound of cooked ham, make small pieces
1 large carrot, sliced into coins
1 tsp. of cumin powder
Shredded cabbage
2 tbs. of butter

Nutritional Value (Per Serving):

Calories – 452 | Fat – 28g | Carbohydrate – 25g | Fiber – 3g | Protein – 21g

Fruit Chicken

Prep Time: 35-40 min. | Serves: 3-4

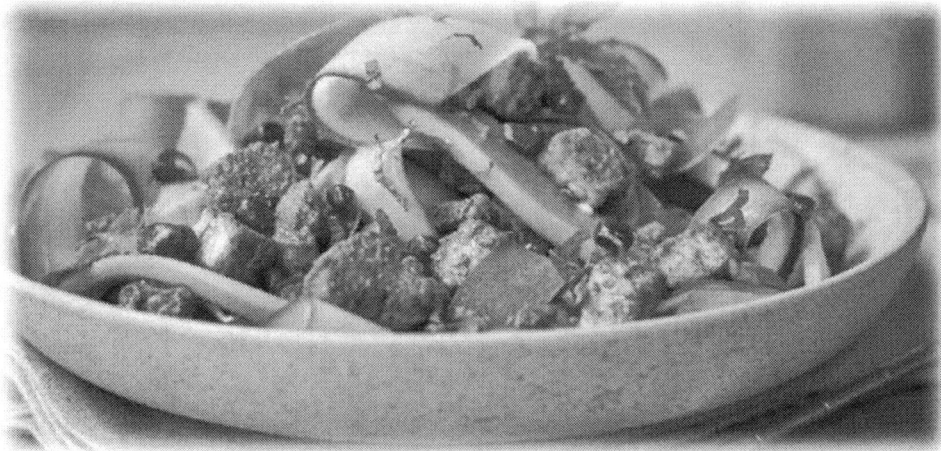

Directions:

- In a bowl of medium size, thoroughly mix all the ingredients and refrigerate overnight.
- Switch on your instant pot. Make sure that your kitchen platform is clean and dry.
- Open the lid and gradually add the mixture in the pot.
- Make sure to lock the lid properly after closing the pot. Also ensure to seal the valve.
- Select "Chicken/Meat" setting from various available options. Adjust cooking time to 25 minutes.
- Allow the mixture to cook under pressure until the timer reads zero.
- Turn off and press "Cancel" setting. Naturally release pressure.
- Open the pot and transfer the mixture to a serving bowl.
- Serve hot with rice.

Ingredients:

½ cup of small papaya pieces
½ cup of raspberry juice
½ cup of orange juice, unsweetened
½ cup of apple pieces
1 pound of chicken breast, skinless, boneless, make small pieces
½ cup of pomegranate juice
1 tsp. of pepper
½ cup of tomato puree, homemade

Nutritional Value (Per Serving):

Calories – 398 | Fat – 6g | Carbohydrate – 48g | Fiber – 4g | Protein – 37.5g

Mushroom Cheese Chicken

Prep Time: 40-45 min. | Serves: 3-4

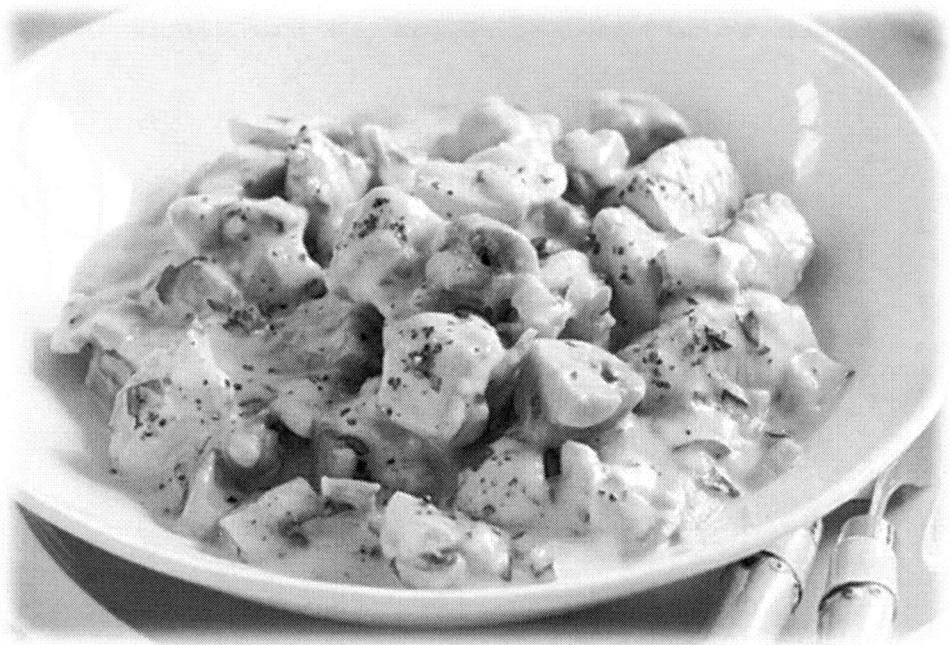

Directions:

- Switch on your instant pot. Make sure that your kitchen platform is clean and dry.
- Select "Saute" setting from various available options.
- Open the pot and add some butter, mushroom and onions; heat for 3 minutes to cook well and soften.
- Add chicken, cheese and parsley; stir to combine.
- Make sure to lock the lid properly after closing the pot. Also ensure to seal the valve.
- Select "Chicken/Meant" setting from various available options. Adjust cooking time to 30 minutes.
- Allow the mixture to cook under pressure until the timer reads zero.
- Turn off and press "Cancel" setting.
- Open the pot and transfer the mixture to a serving bowl.
- Serve hot!

Ingredients:

16 Portobello mushrooms, chopped
4 chicken breasts, skinless, boneless, make cubes
1 ½ cups of cheddar cheese, shredded
2 tbs. of butter
2 tbs. of onions, chopped
1 tbs. of chopped parsley

Nutritional Value (Per Serving):

Calories – 403 | Fat – 12g | Carbohydrate – 13g | Fiber – 4g | Protein – 53.5g

Zucchini Pork Chops

Prep Time: 1 hour 15-20 min. | Serves: 4

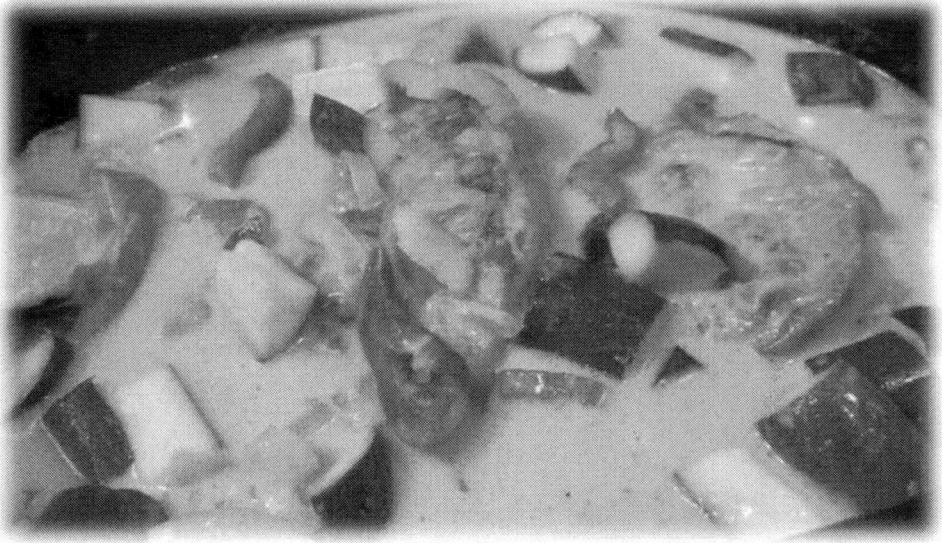

Directions:

- Switch on your instant pot. Make sure that your kitchen platform is clean and dry.
- Select "Saute" setting from various available options.
- Open the pot and add some oil, garlic and onions; heat for 2 minutes to cook well and soften.
- Add zucchini and pork chops.
- Add other ingredients. Mix well.
- Make sure to lock the lid properly after closing the pot. Also ensure to seal the valve.
- Select "Chicken/Meat" setting from various available options. Adjust cooking time to 50 minutes.
- Allow the mixture to cook under pressure until the timer reads zero.
- Turn off and press "Cancel" setting. Naturally release pressure.
- Open the pot and transfer the mixture to a serving bowl.
- Serve hot!

Ingredients:

4 medium zucchini, chopped
4 boneless pork chops, thick cut
¼ cup of cilantro, minced
1 tsp. of almond oil
1 tsp. of minced garlic
1 tbs. of curry powder
¼ tsp. of cayenne pepper
½ cup of onion, diced
½ tsp. of cumin
1 tsp. of spice mix (garam masala)
1 cup of coconut milk

Nutritional Value (Per Serving):

Calories – 411 | Fat – 17g | Carbohydrate – 13.5g | Fiber – 2g | Protein – 34.5g

Mushroom Pepper Curry

Prep Time: 30-35 min. | Serves: 5-6

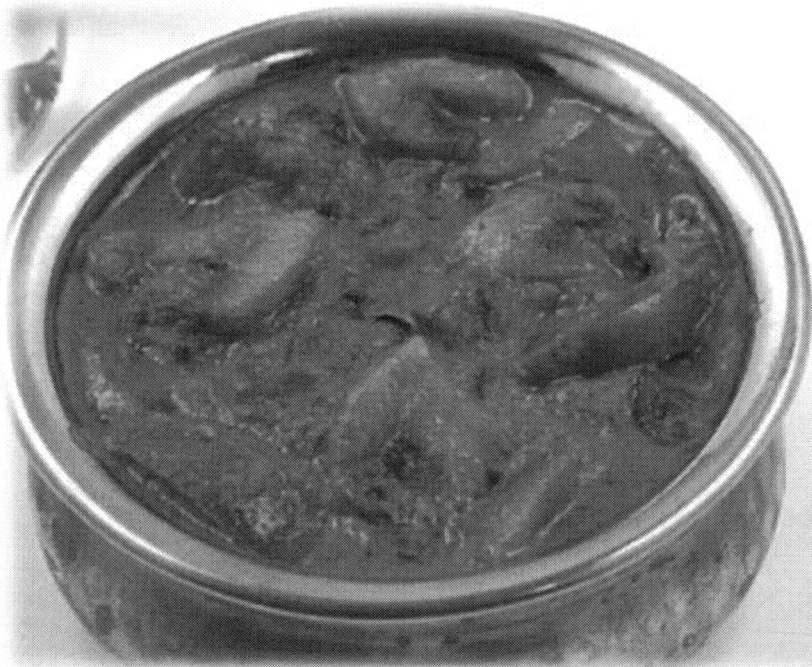

Directions:

- Switch on your instant pot. Make sure that your kitchen platform is clean and dry.
- Open the lid and gradually add all the above mentioned ingredients in the pot. Do not add the sesame seeds.
- Stir the mixture well.
- Make sure to lock the lid properly after closing the pot. Also ensure to seal the valve.
- Select "Stew" setting from various available options. Adjust cooking time to 15 minutes.
- Allow the mixture to cook under pressure until the timer reads zero.
- Turn off and press "Cancel" setting.
- Open the pot and transfer the mixture to a serving bowl.
- Top with the seeds and serve hot!

Ingredients:

¼ cup of green pepper, sliced
2 tbs. of olive oil
8 ounces of Portobello mushrooms, chopped
¼ cup of brown sugar
8 ounces of tomato puree, homemade
¼ cup of cabbage, shredded
½ cup of soy sauce, low-sodium, gluten free
1 tbs. of sesame seeds, toasted

Nutritional Value (Per Serving):

Calories – 545 | Fat – 32g | Carbohydrate – 48.5g | Fiber – 4g | Protein – 13g

Lemon Crabs

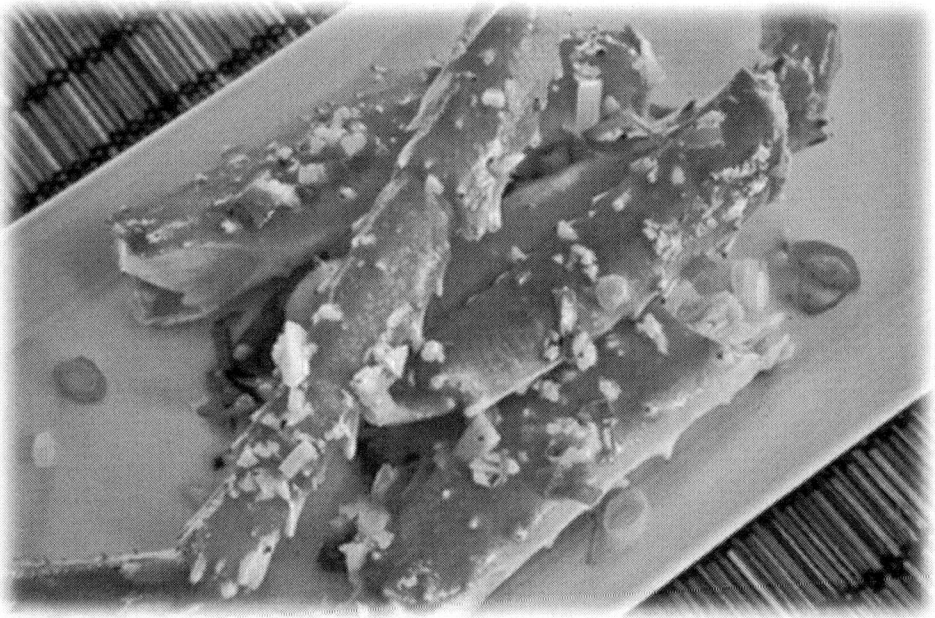

Directions:

- Switch on your instant pot. Make sure that your kitchen platform is clean and dry.
- Pour the water in the pot. Arrange a trivet inside and add crab legs over the trivet.
- Make sure to lock the lid properly after closing the pot. Also ensure to seal the valve.
- Select "Chicken Meat" setting from various available options. Adjust cooking time to 5 minutes.
- Allow the mixture to cook under pressure until the timer reads zero.
- Turn off and press "Cancel" setting.
- Melt butter in a saucepan of medium size; cook and stirring occasionally, until it becomes golden.
- Add the garlic and cook for 1-2 minutes.
- Turn off the heat and mix in lemon juice.
- Add lemon sauce over the crabs and serve!

Ingredients:
1 halved lemon
2 pounds of crab legs, fresh
4 tbs. of butter
1 large garlic clove, minced
1 cup of water

Nutritional Value (Per Serving):
Calories – 342 | Fat – 6g | Carbohydrate – 2g | Fiber – 0g | Protein – 43g

Chapter 4:
Savory Snacks

Wine Potatoes

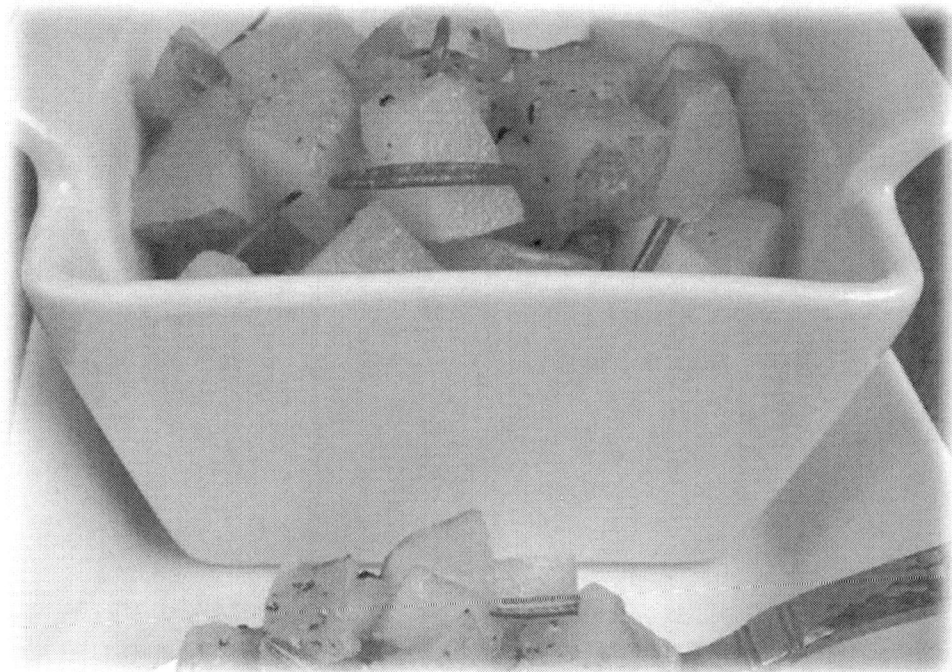

Directions:

- Switch on your instant pot. Make sure that your kitchen platform is clean and dry.
- Select "Saute" setting from various available options.
- Open the pot and add some oil, potatoes, rosemary, salt, and pepper; heat for 4-5 minutes to cook well and soften.
- Mix in some wine and stir a little.
- Make sure to lock the lid properly after closing the pot. Also ensure to seal the valve.
- Select "Risotto" setting from various available options. Adjust cooking time to 8 minutes.
- Allow the mixture to cook under pressure until the timer reads zero.
- Turn off and press "Cancel" setting.
- Open the pot and transfer the mixture to a serving bowl.
- Serve hot!

Ingredients:

4-5 medium diced potatoes, scrubbed
1 cup of Marsala wine
1 sprig rosemary
1 tbs. of olive oil
Pepper and salt to taste

Nutritional Value (Per Serving):

Calories – 276 | Fat – 6g | Carbohydrate – 44.5g | Fiber – 4g | Protein – 12g

Tahini Chickpea Hummus

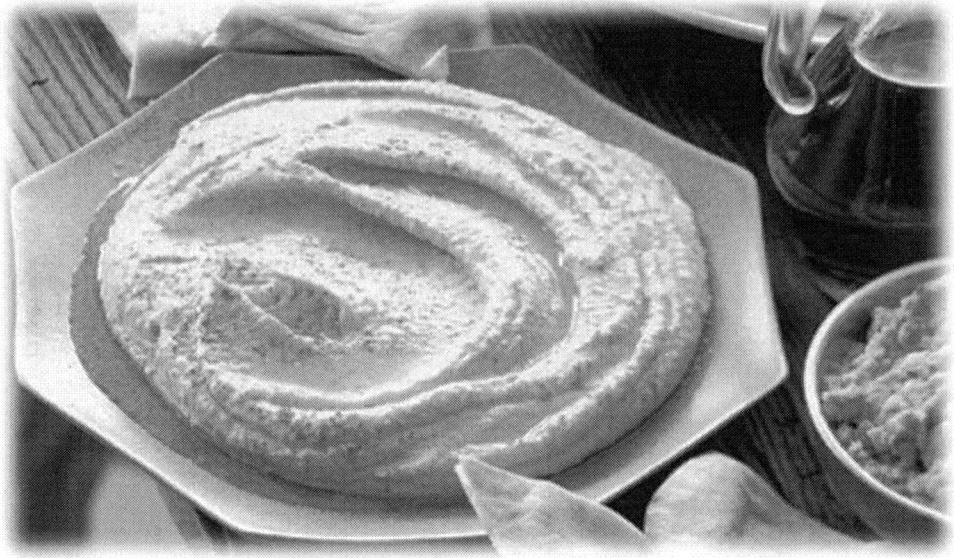

Directions:

- Switch on your instant pot. Make sure that your kitchen platform is clean and dry.
- Open the lid and gradually add 2 tbs. of oil, chickpeas, and water in the pot.
- Make sure to lock the lid properly after closing the pot. Also ensure to seal the valve.
- Select "Chicken/Meat" setting from various available options. Adjust cooking time to 52 minutes.
- Allow the mixture to cook under pressure until the timer reads zero.
- Turn off and press "Cancel" setting.
- Let inside pressure to release naturally; it will take 8-10 minutes for pressure release.
- Open the pot.
- Drain the chickpeas and reserve one cup of the liquid.
- Add the chickpeas in a blender or food processor; add 4 tbs. of olive oil, garlic, lemon juice, salt, paprika, and ¼ cup of liquid.
- Add more liquid for a desired consistency.
- Store in a fridge for up to 4-5 days or serve immediately!

Ingredients:

¼ cup of lemon juice
⅓ cup of tahini
8-ounces of rinsed chickpeas, dried
3 garlic cloves, minced
4 cups of water
6 tbs. of olive oil
1 ½ tsp. of salt
½ tsp. of smoked paprika

Nutritional Value (Per Serving):

Calories – 262 | Fat – 3g | Carbohydrate – 19g | Fiber – 5.5g | Protein – 8g

Chapter 5:
Delicious Desserts

Cream Chocolate

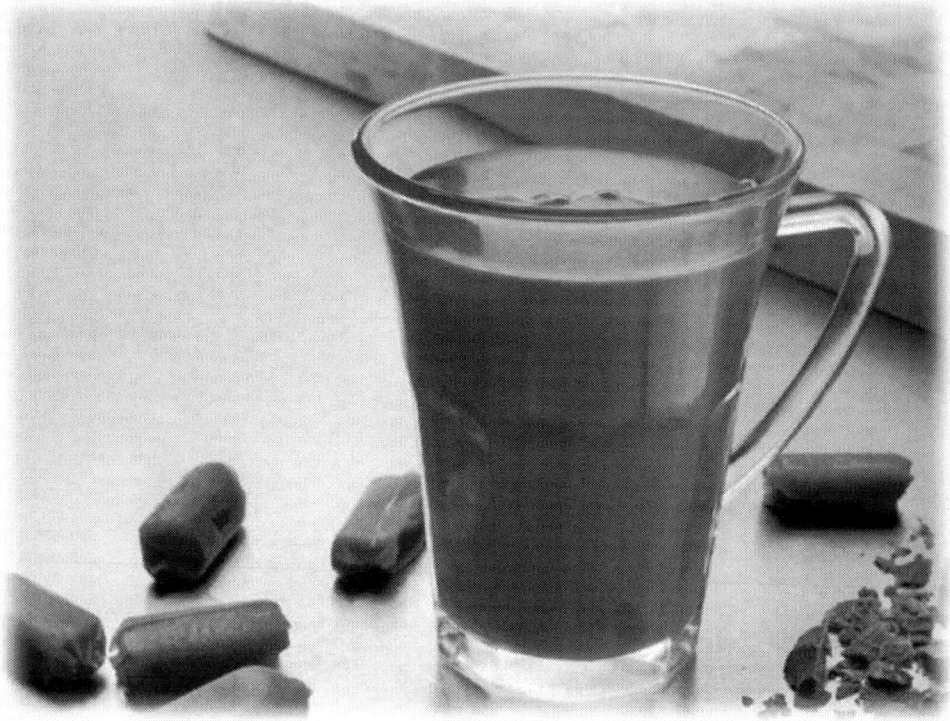

Directions:

- Switch on your instant pot. Make sure that your kitchen platform is clean and dry.
- Pour some water in the pot. Arrange a trivet inside
- In a mug, add chocolate, cream and sugar; put the mug over the trivet.
- Make sure to lock the lid properly after closing the pot. Also ensure to seal the valve.
- Select "Manual" setting from various available options. Adjust cooking time to 2 minutes.
- Allow the mixture to cook under pressure until the timer reads zero.
- Turn off and press "Cancel" setting.
- Stir the mix and serve hot!

Ingredients:

3 1/2 ounces of cream
3 1/2 ounces of chocolate
1 tsp. of sugar
2 cups of water

Nutritional Value (Per Serving):

Calories – 80 | Fat – 5g | Carbohydrate – 6.5g | Fiber – 0g | Protein – 2g

Cinnamon Apples

Prep Time: 10-15 min. | Serves: 5-6

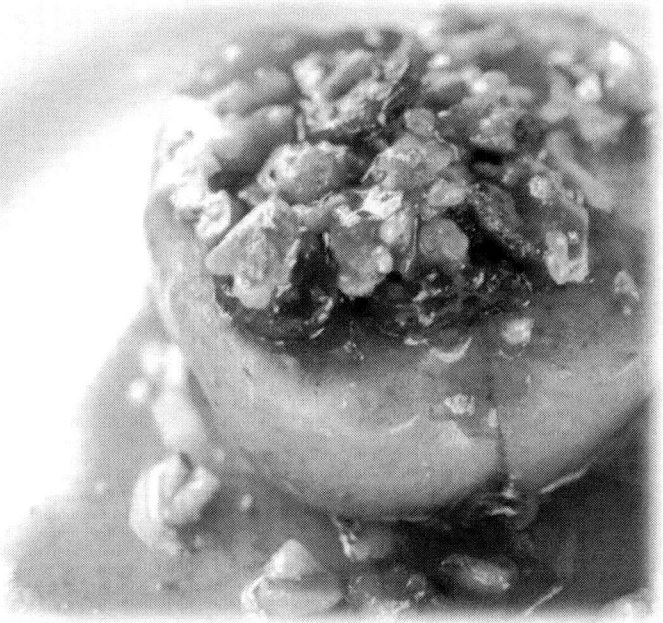

Directions:

Ingredients:
¼ cup of raisins
6 cored apples
1 tsp. of cinnamon
1 cup of red wine
½ cup of brown sugar

- Switch on your instant pot. Make sure that your kitchen platform is clean and dry.
- Open the lid and gradually add apples and then add other ingredients in the pot.
- Make sure to lock the lid properly after closing the pot. Also ensure to seal the valve.
- Select "Manual" setting from various available options. Adjust cooking time to 10 minutes.
- Allow the mixture to cook under pressure until the timer reads zero.
- Turn off and press "Cancel" setting. Naturally release pressure.
- Open the pot and transfer the apples to a serving bowl.
- Top with the pot juice and serve hot!

Nutritional Value (Per Serving):
Calories – 335 | Fat – 2g | Carbohydrate – 62g | Fiber – 9g | Protein – 1g

Yummy Rice Pudding

Prep Time: 10-15 min. | Serves: 2-3

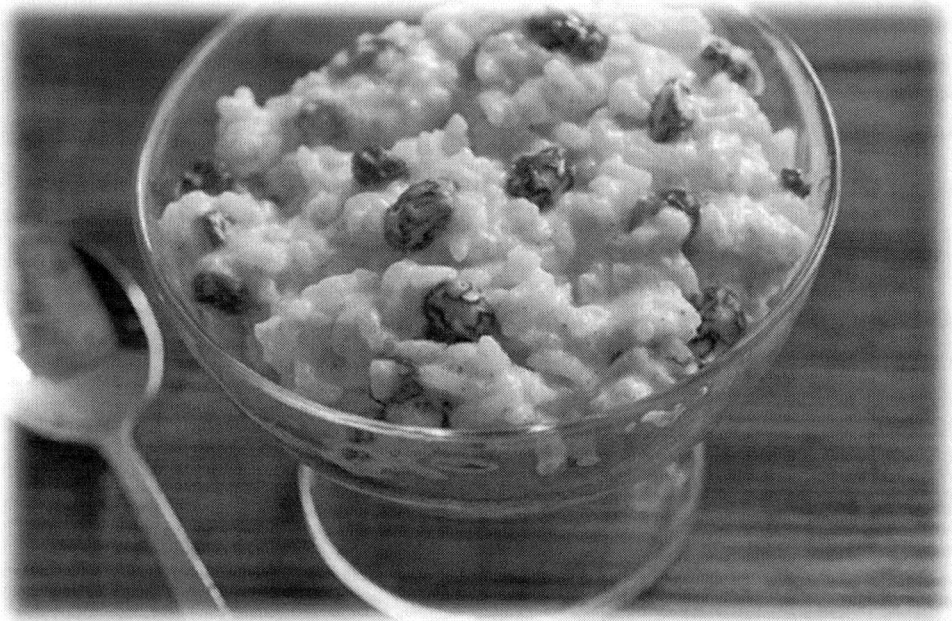

Directions:

- Switch on your instant pot. Make sure that your kitchen platform is clean and dry.
- Open the lid and gradually add some water, salt and rice in the pot.
- Make sure to lock the lid properly after closing the pot. Also ensure to seal the valve.
- Select "Manual" setting from various available options. Adjust cooking time to 3 minutes.
- Allow the mixture to cook under pressure until the timer reads zero.
- Turn off and press "Cancel" setting.
- Open the pot and add just 1 1/2 cups of the milk, sugar. Stir well.
- In a bowl of medium size, thoroughly mix eggs, vanilla, and remaining milk. Whisk and then strain this mixture through a fine strainer.
- Add the mixture into the Pot. Press 'Sauté' and boil the mixture.
- Add the mixture in a serving bowl and add raisins. Stir well.
- Serve hot!

Ingredients:

1 1/2 cups of water
1/2 tsp. of vanilla extract
1 cup of Arborio rice, gluten free
3/4 cup of raisins
1/4 tsp. of salt
2 eggs
2 cups of milk
1/2 cup of sugar

Nutritional Value (Per Serving):

Calories – 535 | Fat – 9g | Carbohydrate – 54.5g | Fiber – 3g | Protein – 15g

Conclusion

Going gluten-free is a healthy lifestyle choice that has been supported and followed by millions of people across the world. Gluten free diet promotes overall health and improves quality of life.

Instant Pot is your true kitchen companion that helps you enjoy your favorite gluten-free meals along with preserving their unique nutritional balance. There are multiple benefits of making use of an Instant Pot. It is easy to operate; easy to clean and compact to fit in little space in your kitchen.

The book aims at delivering the most versatile collection of 40 Instant Pot Gluten Free recipes to maintain one's optimum health. We are ascertain that the versatile recipes covered in the book will help all its readers to make heavenly delicious meals, breakfast, snacks, appetizers, and desserts at home and enjoy with your whole family. You can also experiment with the recipes by adding your favorite ingredients and create the own customized recipe.

Finally, if you enjoyed this dedicated book, please take a few minutes of your valuable time to share your views and suggestion at -- email address --. It'd be greatly appreciated!

Thank you and have a great time enjoying these delicious recipes!

Happy Cooking!

Made in the USA
Columbia, SC
13 November 2018